TAPE IT & MAKE IT

Richela Fabian Morgan

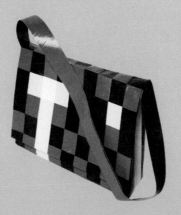

101 CRAFT ADVENTURES WITH DUCT TAPE

Search Press

D0620322

MERTHYR TYDFIL
LIBRARIES

Bertrams	16/10/2012
745.572MOR	£9.99

A QUINTET BOOK

Published in 2012 by Search Press Ltd
Wellwood
North Farm Road
Tunbridge Wells
Kent TN2 3DR
United Kingdom

Copyright © 2012 Quintet Publishing Limited

ISBN: 978-1-84448-912-1

This book may not be reproduced in whole
or in part, in any form or by any means, electronic or
mechanical, including photocopying, recording or by any information
storage and retrieval system known or hereafter invented, without
the prior permission of the copyright holder.

Velcro® is a registered trademark of Velcro Industries B. V.

Duck™ brand tape is a trademark of Shurtech Brands, LLC. This book
is in no way associated with or endorsed by Shurtech Brands, LLC.

QTT.DUCT

This book was conceived, designed, and produced by
Quintet Publishing Limited
The Old Brewery
6 Blundell Street
London N7 9BH
UK

Project Editor: Ross Fulton
Consultant: Megan Hiller
Design: rawshock.co.uk
Photography: Simon Pask
Lead Crafter: Danielle Hall
Assistant Crafters: Gareth Butterworth, Ivana Prauge
Art Director: Michael Charles
Editorial Director: Donna Gregory
Publisher: Mark Searle

Printed in China by 1010 Printing International Limited

9 8 7 6 5 4 3 2 1

Contents

INTRODUCTION

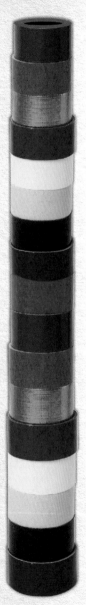

I WAS WALKING DOWN THE STREET ONE SUNNY AFTERNOON, handbag slung halfway up one forearm, sunglasses in place and hair properly coiffed. You could say that I was having an Audrey Hepburn moment, and I felt all eyes on me. Trying to fully realize the role I had imagined for myself, I stopped by each shop's window and then casually sauntered until something caught my attention. In the reflection of the stationery shop's window, I noticed that people were not looking at me. They were looking at my handbag.

I would have been jealous of my handbag if it were not for the fact that I actually made it – yes, me and my two crafty hands. And not only did I make it, I used (insert trumpet blasts here) duct tape. My handbag is a red, white and black duct tape confection finessed into a faux Burberry tartan. It is constantly mistaken for patent leather, and often will draw an admirer's touch. 'Wow', this stranger would say, 'that's cool'! And I had to admit, it really was cool.

Ya gotta love duct tape.

Duct tape has been around since the 1940s, when it was originally developed as an adhesive for ammunition cases during World War II. Because of its water resistant qualities, the military also used it for quick fixes on jeeps and firearms. It eventually found its way into hardware stores, where plumbers and builders gave it its current name.

Nowadays, duct tape is ubiquitous. Besides a hardware store, you can find a roll of the good stuff in an office supply shop, an arts 'n' crafts store, a grocery store, and even a chemist – all places that one would certainly not associate with malfunctioning ducts. So why are these places stocking up on duct tape?

The answer is: duct tape is the new black – and not just in the fashion sense. You can make just about anything with it, from accessories to home decorations. Need a cool luggage tag? Make it out of duct tape. What about a toy boat? Duct tape is the answer. And you can still use it for repairs, from ducts to pillows to furniture. But instead of noticing a slapdash quality to the mend, you'll nod in appreciation of the fine handiwork.

Neither can you only get it in the basic silver colour: duct tape is available in all primary colours, secondary colours, metallic colours, day-glow colours, animal prints, tie-dye prints, superhero prints, psychedelic prints, and, of course, camouflage. I've seen all of these varieties in a single aisle of a craft store, solely dedicated to duct tape.

From the stuff of quick military repairs to the material du jour of hip crafters, duct tape has come a long, long way. Let's get started.

YOUR WORKSPACE, CLEANING AND STORAGE

Duct tape is a gummy, sticky medium, and it can be quite unforgiving once you make a mistake. A smooth surface that is less porous than wood – like a Formica or melamine tabletop – is perfect to work on. It needs to be dust-free, so wipe it down with a damp cloth before you start work.

After working on your project, throw away any excess tape and properly clean the blades of the craft knife and scissors. The best way to remove the sticky gunk that builds up on some surfaces is to wipe them down with a dab of mineral oil or petroleum jelly. Store all rolls of tape in a transparent bin with a lid. This will enable you to see what colours and patterns you have without opening the bin, and keeps the tape dust-free.

NECESSARY TOOLS

The following tools are used in every project in this book:
- Self-healing cutting mat, size 30 cm x 90 cm (12 in x 36 in)
- Craft knife (size 10), and extra blades
- Metal ruler with cork backing, 30 cm (12 in) long
- Metal ruler with cork backing, 60 cm (24 in) long
- Scissors
- Detail scissors

Keep these on your worktable, ready to be used at any moment. Any extra tools required are listed in each project's 'Additional Tools' section.

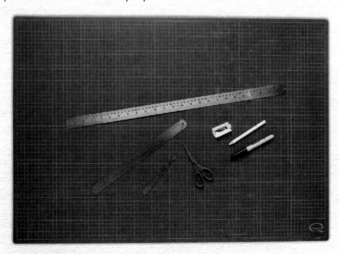

COLOURS AND PATTERNS

Any colours of duct tape can be used for the projects in this book, not just those suggested in the instructions. If you can't get your hands on some patterned tapes, like zebra-print or camouflage, then that's all the more reason to be bold and creative in your colour choices and combinations.

CREATING DUCT TAPE FABRICS

'SQUARING UP'

When making duct tape fabrics, you will need to 'square up' the edges. This means that the edges of the fabric should be neatly trimmed using a metal ruler and craft knife, and that the edges should be perpendicular to each other. Use the grid on the self-healing cutting mat to ensure that each corner is exactly 90 degrees.

AVOIDING BUBBLES OR BUMPS

It is important to clean the cutting mat before laying down any tape. Wipe down the mat with a damp cloth; wipe again with a dry cloth. Run your hand across it to check for any stuck-on debris and wipe again if needed.

VARIETIES OF DUCT TAPE FABRIC

One-Sided Layered Fabric

For this fabric, the reverse side will remain sticky unless a thin cotton handkerchief, bandana or polyester scarf is affixed to it to act as a lining.

1. Unwind the roll of tape across the surface of a cutting mat to the desired length. Cut off this strip with scissors.
2. Lay another strip of tape across the cutting mat, overlapping the first strip by 3 mm (⅛ in). Repeat until you reach the desired overall size.
3. Square up the fabric. From the top right corner, gently peel off the tape across the diagonal to prevent the pieces from coming apart.

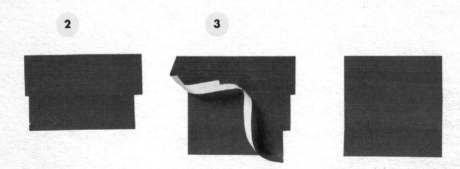

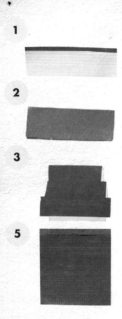

Double-Sided Layered Fabric

This duct tape fabric is slightly thicker than the single layer. For a two-tone look, use two different colors for the fabric's front and back sides – this not only looks more playful, it also allows you to make your project reversible.

1. Cut a piece of duct tape and place it on the cutting mat, sticky side facing up. Fold down the top edge to make a 6 mm (¼ in) border.
2. Lay the second strip of tape sticky side down, across the first strip so they overlap by 6 mm (¼ in) on both their top and bottom edges.
3. Flip it over so that the sticky side of the bottom strip is facing up. Lay another strip of tape, sticky side down, across the bottom strip, overlapping by the same measure. Repeat this step until you reach your desired height.
4. Once you've reached the desired height, flip the fabric over so that the last strip is at the bottom, with the sticky side facing up.
5. Fold over the bottom edge so that the sticky side is completely covered, then square up the fabric.

Woven Fabric

This simple up-and-over technique allows you to create checkered patterns, and also Piet Mondrian–type squares. Or if you use a single colour, the fabric takes on a more tactile quality which really transforms the duct tape into something else entirely.

1. Lay strips of tape horizontally across the cutting mat, sticky side down. Leave a slight gap between each strip, but make sure that each is no greater than 1.5 mm (¹⁄₁₆ in).
2. Starting on the right edge, pull up every other strip and gently double them back on themselves. Then place a strip of duct tape vertically down, across those strips that remain stuck down. Replace the pulled-up horizontal strips on top of the vertical strip.
3. Pull the alternate horizontal strips up, starting on the right side and working toward the left. Vertically place another strip of duct tape to the immediate left edge of the first vertical strip, as close to it as possible without actually touching. Then, replace the lifted horizontal strips on the top of the new vertical strip. Repeat this step until you reach the desired size of the fabric.
4. Gently pry up the fabric's lower right corner, and pull it up off the cutting mat in a diagonal motion toward its upper left corner.
5. Put down the fabric with its sticky side facing upward. Cover the sticky surface with a thin cotton material, like an old t-shirt or bandana. Use your hands to smooth out any air bubbles, then square-up the edges of the fabric, and flip it over to reveal the front side of the finished woven fabric.

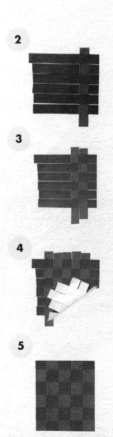

CHAPTER 1:

Accessories

When it comes to accessories, duct tape can either be a last-minute lifesaver or a well-executed piece of wearable art. Because of the patterns and colours that are now available, duct tape can resemble absolutely anything rather than that utilitarian adhesive of yesteryear.

Most of the following projects are inspired by pop culture as well as the indomitable attitude of being young and in the moment. But those who are forever 21 can also enjoy the whimsy of these bright, bold and beautiful playthings.

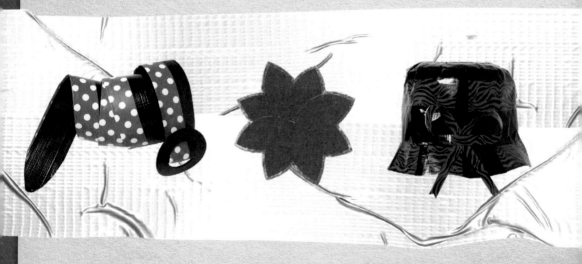

PROPERTY OF MERTHYR
TYDFIL PUBLIC LIBRARIES

Materials

» Hot pink duct tape
» Black and white
  zebra print duct tape
» Masking tape

Additional Tools

» White grease pencil

1. Feather

1 Cut one strip of hot pink duct tape and one strip of zebra print duct tape, each of them at least 22.5 cm (9 in) long.

2 Flip the zebra print over so the sticky side is facing up. Carefully place the hot pink strip on top of it, aligning the edges. With the hot pink side facing up, hold the combined strip in place with masking tape. Using the white grease pencil and metal ruler, measure and draw a line lengthwise down the middle of the strip. Using the craft knife, cut out the outer shape of a feather. Then cut slits on the left and right sides directed downwards at a 45-degree angle. Be sure to not cut beyond the white border in the middle.

3 With your fingers loosen the slits and fluff it out. Then, using the detail scissors, cut more, finer slits into the left and right sides, making sure to cut through both the pink and zebra-print layers of duct tape.

4 Again, loosen the slits and fluff it out with your fingers.

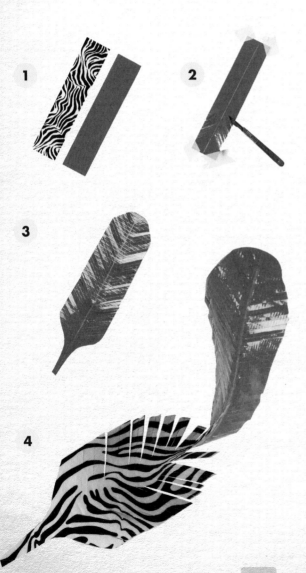

1

2

3

4

2. Headband

Materials

» Red duct tape
» Black and white zebra print duct tape
» 22.5 cm (9 in.) strip of elastic band
» Two glue dots

1 Cut a 25 cm (10 in) strip of red duct tape. Fold it vertically in half so that the edges line up. You should now have a double-sided strip that measures 12.75 cm (5 in).

2 Cut a strip of red duct tape around 12.75 cm (5 in) long and 1.25 cm (½ in) wide. Pinch the double-sided strip in the middle and wrap one end of the 1.25-cm (½-in) wide strip of red duct tape once around it, leaving the tail of the 1.25-cm (½-in) wide strip free. This is the bow.

3 Cut a 30 cm (12 in) strip of black and white zebra duct tape. Fold it in half lengthwise. This is the main body of the headband.

4 Place the bow approximately 10 cm (4 in) from the left edge of the headband, measuring from the middle of the bow. Use the remaining tail of the 1.25-cm (½-in) wide red strip to wrap the bow around the headband.

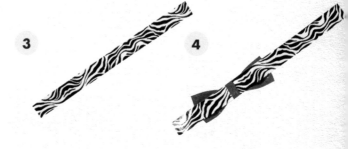

5 Flip the headband over so the back is facing upward. Put a glue dot on one end of the elastic band and then affix it to one end of the headband. Fold the corners of the headband ends inward and hold them in place with a small piece of black and white zebra duct tape.

6 Repeat Step 5 on the other end of the headband.

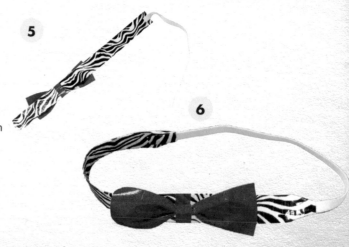

3. Two-finger Ring

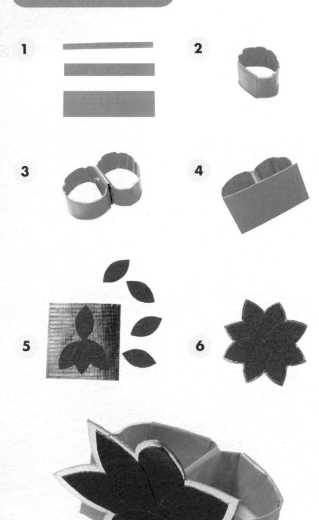

1 Cut a 17.5 cm (7 in) length of lime green duct tape. Cut it in half lengthwise, then fold one of these halves over lengthwise.

2 Wrap the strip around your middle finger and measure the circumference; add around 3 mm (1/8 in) of slack and cut off any excess. Hold the strip together with a piece of lime green duct tape.

3 Repeat Step 2, using the excess part of the strip to make a second ring. Attach both rings to each other with a piece of lime green duct tape.

4 Take a 5 cm (2 in) strip of lime green duct tape and fold it into itself, sticky sides facing inward. Trim this down to a 2.5 x 3.75 cm (1 in x 1½ in) rectangle. Place glue dots on top of the two rings, then affix the rectangle on top, making sure to centre it on top of the rings.

5 Cut a 10 cm (4 in) strip of silver chrome duct tape, fold it over on itself and trim it down to a 5 cm x 5 cm (2 in x 2 in) square. Then cut eight 2.5-cm (1-in) pointed ellipses from red duct tape.

6 Arrange these ellipses onto the silver square in a flower formation. Trim the silver tape so there is a 1.5 mm (1/16 in) border around the red flower. Attach the red flower to the ring with glue dots.

Materials

» Lime green duct tape
» Red duct tape
» Silver chrome duct tape
» Glue dots

4. Two-tone Bracelet

Materials

» Royal blue duct tape
» Silver chrome duct tape

1 Begin to make a 25 cm (10 in) long double-sided layered fabric (see page 9) using only three strips. Use royal blue duct tape for the first and second strips, and silver chrome duct tape for the third strip. Leave the final, silver strip open and unfinished.

2 Flip it over so that the silver strip is along the top edge with the sticky side face-up. Align the bottom edge with one of the horizontal grid lines on the cutting mat. Then carefully fold down the top edge so that the height measures 6.25 cm (2½ in) and lines up with the appropriate horizontal grid line on the cutting mat.

3 Flip over again. Fold the entire piece lengthwise so that the overall height is 3.75 cm (1½ in). Wrap it around your wrist and measure the necessary circumference: it should be loose enough to remove, but tight enough that it can't slip off. Cut off the excess part.

4 Cut a piece of silver chrome duct tape measuring 2.5 cm (1 in) wide. Use this to seal the join between the two ends of the bracelet, with the strip's long sides running parallel to the join.

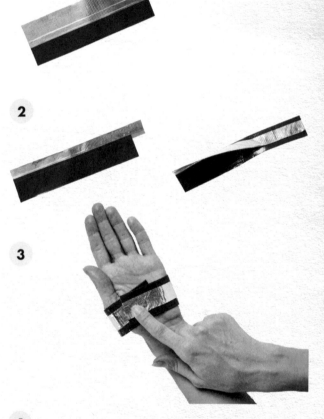

Materials

» Blue and purple tie dye duct tape
» Scrap paper

Additional Tools

» Pencil
» White grease pencil

5. Fingerless Gloves

1 Place your hand on top of the scrap paper and trace an outline for a fingerless glove, tracing around your hand but stopping just above the first knuckle of each finger, and just below your wrist. Leave a border of at least 7.5 mm (¼ in) on the left and right edges. Cut out this stencil with a craft knife.

2 Make two double-sided layered fabrics measuring 27.5 cm x 20.5 cm (11 in x 8 in).

3 Trace the glove pattern twice on each of the two fabric pieces. Then cut out all four glove parts from the fabric.

4 Take a 50 cm (20 in) strip of duct tape and cut it lengthwise into smaller 1.25-cm (½-in) wide strips.

5 Take two of the glove pieces and place them on the cutting mat. Place the remaining two glove pieces on top, aligning the edges. Use the 1.25-cm (½-in) wide strips to seal up the outside edges (along the pinky finger) plus the inner edges between the thumb and forefinger. Then seal up approximately 5 cm (2 in) of the inside edge, starting at the wrist and proceeding toward the thumb. Leave the rest of the inside edge open.

6 Turn the gloves inside-out and repeat Step 5 to seal the outer seams and complete the gloves.

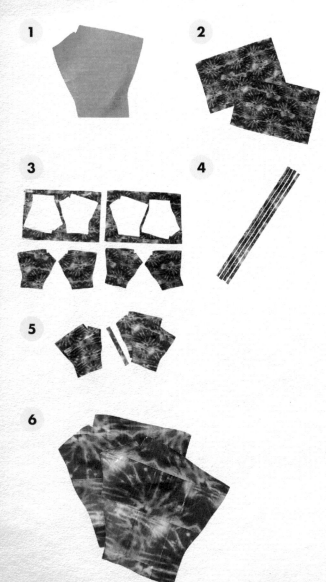

1

2

3

4

5

6

6. Belt

Materials

» Pink and white polka
  dot duct tape
» Black duct tape
» "O" style belt buckle

1 Take a 60 cm (24 in) strip of pink and white polka dot duct tape and, with its sticky side facing upward, fold down the top edge to make a 6 mm (¼ in) border (as though making a double-sided fabric, see page 9). Set it aside.

2 Repeat Step 1, but before closing up the edge, place the first piece on top so that it overlaps by 1.25 cm (½ in), and fold the top edge of the second piece down over it. You should now have one long piece that measures at least 108 cm (43 in).

3 Add a strip of black duct tape across the entire 108 cm (43 in) length of the polka dot piece, covering and overlapping its exposed sticky side.

4 Flip over and place a second strip of black duct tape lengthwise across the exposed sticky edge of the previous strip of black duct tape.

5 Flip over so the sticky side of the second strip is facing up and along the top edge. Fold the top edge over and downward, making the belt 7.5 cm (3 in) wide.

6 Round the corners of one end of the belt using detail scissors.

7 Attach the "O" style belt buckle to the other end of the belt, using a strip of black duct tape.

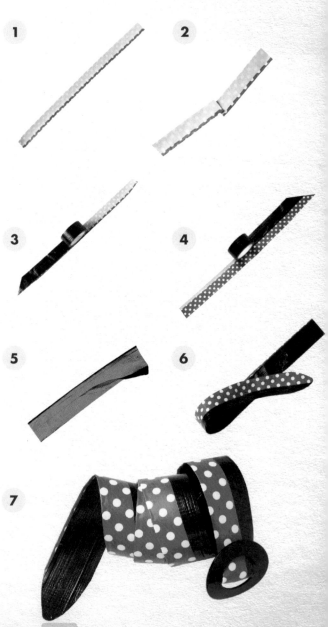

Materials

» Hot pink duct tape
» Teal duct tape
» Small piece of scrap paper, at least 7.5 cm (3 in) square
» 8.75 cm (3½ in) hair clip
» Glue dots

Additional Tools

» White grease pencil

1

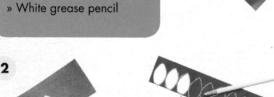

7. Flower Hair Clip

1 Cut two 50 cm (20 in) lengths of duct tape – one teal, one hot pink. Combine them with both sticky sides facing inward, aligning their edges.

2 On scrap paper, draw a flower petal template 3.75 cm (1½ in) high and 2.5 cm (1 in) wide, with a pointed top edge and a flat bottom edge. Cut it out, then trace it onto the double-sided duct tape strip twenty times in a row. Cut out the petals.

3 Fold one petal vertically, with the pink side facing inward. Add a glue dot to one outer side of the petal's base. Fold another petal vertically and attach it to the first petal at the base. Add another glue dot to the outside petal's base.

4 Repeat Step 3 until all petals are attached, then affix the final petal to the first to form a circle.

5 Cut two 5 cm (2 in) squares of duct tape, one hot pink and the other teal, and affix one on top of the other with both sticky sides facing inward. Place a few glue dots onto the centre of the square's hot pink side and place the flower on top, its teal side facing downward.

6 Affix the hair clip's flat edge to the back of the flower with glue dots at a 45-degree angle. Add a small piece of teal duct tape across the clip's flat edge to secure it to the flower.

2

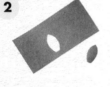
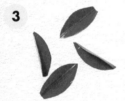

3

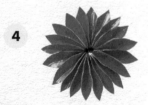
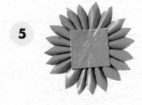

4

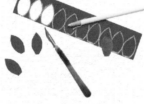

5

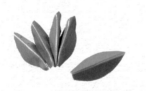

6

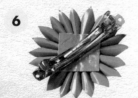
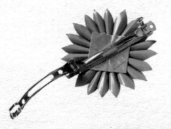

8. Striped Apron

Materials

» Pink and white polka dot duct tape
» White duct tape

Additional Tools

» Thin black marker

1 Make a striped double-sided layered fabric, alternating between plain white and pink-and-white polka dot tape strips, and measuring 35 cm x 60 cm (14 in x 24 in). Square up the sides. Then place a strip of polka dot duct tape across the fabric's top edge.

2 Flip the fabric over from left to right. Place another strip of polka dot duct tape across the top edge, and make another double-sided layer fabric of equal width, again alternating between white and polka dot tape strips. Continue until the second piece is 35 cm (14 in) high.

3 Fold the combined fabric vertically in half. On the top edge make two marks 12.75 cm (5 in) outward from the central fold on either side. Use a black marker to draw curved diagonal lines from these marks to either end of the strip joining the two fabrics, leaving overhanging tabs around 2 cm (¾ in) wide. Cut along these lines with a craft knife.

4 To create ties for the back, fold a length of white duct tape into thirds lengthwise to form a thin rope, and cut off two 30.5 cm (12 in) pieces. Attach one end of each piece to the apron's sides with glue dots, then cover the joins with strips of white duct tape.

5 To create a loop for the top, cut another 60 cm (24 in) rope and attach each end to the apron's top corners with glue dots. Cover each end with a strip of white duct tape.

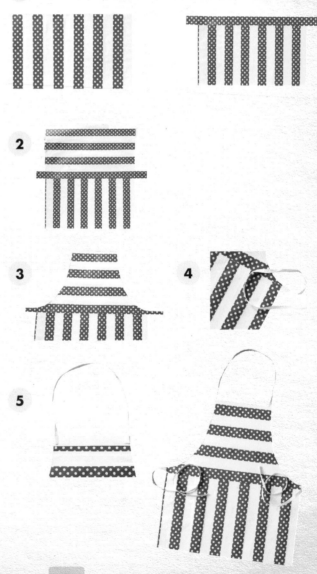

Materials

» Teal duct tape
» Silver duct tape
» An old waistcoat
» Brown paper

Additional Tools

» Pencil
» Scissors
» White grease pencil

9. Waistcoat

1 Trace the outline of the back, left and right sides of an old waistcoat onto brown paper. Cut these stencils out with scissors.

2 Make a double-sided layered fabric, one side teal and the other silver, Trace the stencil for the back of the waistcoat onto this fabric's teal side with a grease pencil, then cut out the shape with a craft knife.

3 Make double-sided fabrics for the waistcoat's left and right sides, both teal on one side and silver on the other. Trace the stencils onto the teal sides of the fabrics and cut them out.

4 Set the back piece of the waistcoat down with its silver side facing upward, then place the left and right pieces on top with their silver sides facing downward. Line up the edges. Cut two pieces of silver tape 2.5 cm (1 in) wide and 5 cm (2 in) high and use them to attach the top edges of the waistcoat's side pieces to the top edges of the back piece.

5 Cut a 15 cm (6 in) strip of silver duct tape, then halve it lengthwise. Use it to join the side edges of the waistcoat from the inside.

6 Cut a 30 cm (12 in) strip of teal duct tape, and cut this lengthwise into three 1.25-cm (½-in) wide strips. Use these strips to seal the outer seams on the top and sides.

7 To create the Peace Sign sticker, see page 50.

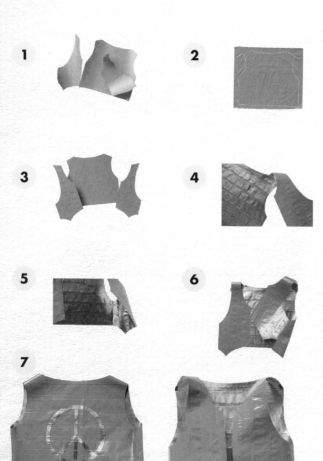

10. Bucket Hat

Materials

» Black duct tape
» Hot pink zebra print duct tape
» Scrap paper, at least 8 in. x
  20.5 cm x 20.5 cm (8 in)
» Glue dots

Additional Tools

» Protractor
» Pencil
» White grease pencil

1 Make a double-sided layered fabric measuring 55 cm x 12.75 cm (22 in. x 5 in). Alternate between the black and the hot pink zebra print duct tape to create stripes of various heights. Trim the edges, then cut triangular indents into the top edge of the fabric about 2.5 cm (1 in) wide and 1.25 cm (½ in) deep, spacing them about 1.25 cm (½ in) apart.

2 Use a protractor and pencil to draw a circle with a 8.75 cm (3½ in) radius on the scrap paper. Cut out this shape. Make a black double-sided layer fabric at least 20.5 cm (8 in) square. Trace the circle template with the white grease pencil, then cut it out of the fabric.

3 Attach the circular top of the hat to the first rectangular piece by folding the indented flaps inward and attaching them to the inside of the circle with small pieces of duct tape.

4 Once the side of the hat is attached to the top edge all the way round, place the hat on top of your head for sizing. If you need to make it wider, pull apart the seam of the side piece and add a strip of black duct tape to the gap; if not, simply close up the seam with black duct tape on both the inside and outside, and trim any excess duct tape from the bottom.

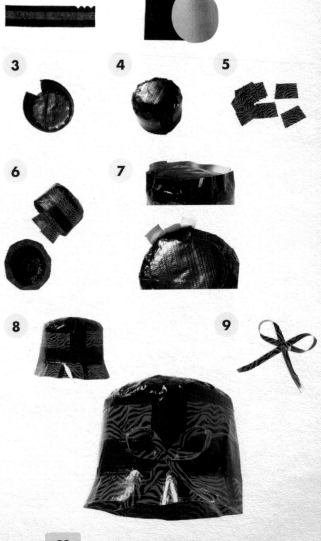

5 Cut at least ten trapezoid pieces of pink zebra print tape, each measuring 7.5 cm (3 in) along the top edge, 6.25 cm (2½ in) along the bottom edge and 5 cm (2 in) high.

6 Attach the trapezoid pieces to the hat's inside bottom edge using 1.25-cm (½-in) wide strips of black duct tape. Attach the sides of each trapezoid piece to the others on the inside bottom edge with black tape.

7 Cut a 60 cm (24 in) strip of black duct tape. Wrap it around the top edge of the hat, leaving half of its sticky side exposed. Cut vertical slits into this strip to create tabs, then fold each of these tabs over the top edge of the hat.

8 Use strips of black tape, 5.75 cm (2¼ in) long and 1.25 cm (½ in) wide, to seal the joins between the trapezoid pieces of the hat's brim. Then cut a strip of black tape 60 cm (24 in) long and 1.25 cm (½ in) high, and use it to cover the seam between the body of the hat and its brim.

9 Take a 50 cm (20 in) strip of hot pink zebra duct tape, and cut it in half lengthwise. Fold one of these halves in on itself lengthwise, creating a double-sided strip. Cross the strip 4 in. (10 cm) from its ends, then pull the middle downward behind it to form the bow, holding the shape in place with glue dots. Cut forked points into each end of the bow. Use more glue dots to attach the bow to the back of the hat.

Materials

» Leopard print duct tape
» Silver chrome duct tape
» Black duct tape
» Standard men's necktie (for reference only)

11. Striped Necktie

1 Make a double-sided layered fabric measuring 50 to 55 cm (20 to 22 in) wide and 30 cm (12 in) high. Alternate the stripes starting with leopard print duct tape, then black, then silver. Square up the edges.

2 Use a long metal ruler and craft knife to cut the fabric at a 45-degree angle, starting from one of the corners. Cut strips along the same angle that measure 7.5 cm (3 in) wide.

3 Connect the strips together with duct tape, matching the sequence of stripes.

4 Trim each end of the tie into triangular points with 90-degree apexes. Your tie is now ready to wear (assuming you know how to knot it).

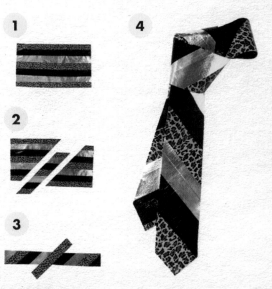

CHAPTER 2:

Housewares

Let's be honest: when you think of duct tape and housewares, you really don't picture anything sleek or well-intentioned.

I felt the same way for a very long time. When I was a kid, that ubiquitous roll of duct tape in the utility drawer was used to fix the rips in the vinyl seats of our kitchen chairs. It also somehow made its way onto broken hoover hoses and the nearly severed electrical cords of not only the iron but the toaster as well. Quick repair jobs were not the equivalent of high design.

The following projects will change your mind about the possibilities of duct tape around the house. From a place to hold your plastic bags to decorative lettering for a mantel or bookshelf, duct tape can add a little pizzazz to an otherwise ordinary corner of your home.

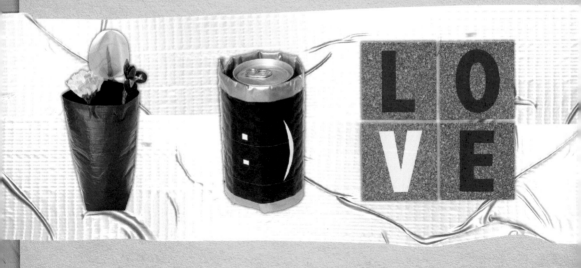

Materials

» Royal blue duct tape
» Black duct tape
» Silver duct tape
» Glue dots

Additional Tools

» Four binder clips

12. Loose Coin Holder

1 Cut eight 28 cm (9 in) strips of duct tape, four royal blue and four black, and cut each in half lengthwise to make sixteen in total.

2 Make a woven fabric using the sixteen strips (see the instructions on page 9).

3 Gently pry the fabric up in a diagonal motion and lay it face down on the cutting mat. Cover its sticky side with silver duct tape, overlapping it by 1.5 mm (¹⁄₁₆ in) on each side.

4 Flip the fabric over and square up the sides. There should be a 1.25 cm (½ in) border around the checkered pattern.

5 Cut two 28 cm (9 in) strips of silver duct tape, then cut each in half lengthwise. Use these to cover the 1.25 cm (½ in) border around each side. Flip the fabric over and fold the overlapping strips onto the back side. Trim the corners of any excess duct tape, then flip it back over.

6 Fold all four of the fabric's sides upward, then pinch its four corners with binder clips to hold this box shape in place.

7 Secure the box shape by opening each corner and placing glue dots inside the crease. Pinch the corners so that the glue dots adhere to both sides of the duct tape.

1
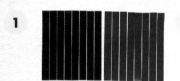

2

3
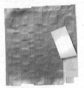

4

5

6
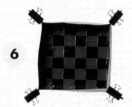

7
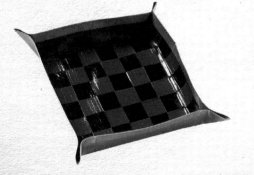

13. Picture Frame

Materials

» Pink/yellow/orange tie-dye duct tape
» White duct tape
» Piece of cardboard measuring 22.5 cm x 30 cm (9 in x 12 in)

Additional Tools

» Pencil or pen
» Masking tape

1 Make a double-sided layered fabric measuring 22.5 cm (9 in) wide by 30 cm (12 in) high using pink/yellow/orange tie-dye duct tape.

2 With the fabric in the portrait position, draw an inner rectangle measuring 13.75 cm (5 in) wide by 17.5 cm (7 in) high. This will create a border 6.25 cm (2½ in) high at the top and bottom edges, and 5 cm (2 in) wide at the sides. Use the metal ruler and craft knife to cut out and remove the inner rectangle. Place the photo face down on the frame shape which remains, centred inside the cut-out area. Hold the photo in place with masking tape.

3 Flip over and place the frame and photo on top of the cardboard, which will be used as the back part of the frame. Hold both sides together with strips of white duct tape at each of the four corners in a 45-degree angle.

1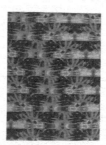

2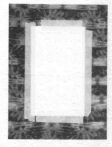

3

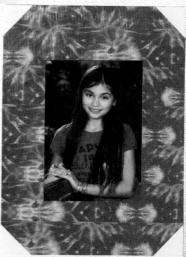

Materials

» 30 cm (12 in) square cork tile
» Red duct tape
» White duct tape

Additional Tools

» Computer and printer

14. Decorative Letters

1 Cut the cork tile into four equal 15 cm (6 in) squares. Set aside.

2 To create the "LOVE" stencil, use a simple word processing application such as Microsoft Word on your computer. Type the word "LOVE" (all capital letters) in a 500-point sans-serif font like Abadi MT Condensed Extra Bold, Arial Black, Futura Bold or Helvetica. Print it out, using two sheets of paper if necessary.

3 Place two 15 cm (6 in) strips of red duct tape on the cutting mat, so that they overlap lengthwise by 1.5 to 3 mm ($\frac{1}{16}$ to $\frac{1}{8}$ in). Place the "L" over it. Carefully cut out the letter with the craft knife. Be sure to cut through both the paper and the duct tape below it.

4 Remove the excess duct tape from the "L." Gently pry up a corner of the letter with the craft knife and remove it by hand. Place the letter in the centre of one of the cork squares.

5 Repeat Steps 3 and 4 with the other letters (O, V and E).

1

2

LOVE

3

4

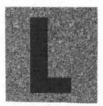

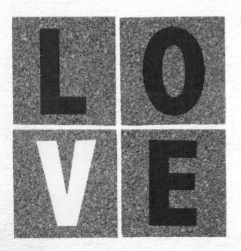

15. Plastic Bag Dispenser

Materials

» Yellow duct tape
» White duct tape
» 91.5 cm (3 ft) of nylon rope
» Glue dots

1 Make a yellow double-sided layered fabric measuring 51 cm x 38 cm (20 in x 15 in), but using white tape for the third and fourth strips from the top.

2 Bring the top and bottom edges together to create a cylinder, and seal the seam with a strip of white duct tape. Turn the cylinder inside-out, and seal the seam again.

3 Cut two 23 cm (9 in) strips of white duct tape, and cut one in half lengthwise. Place one half-strip along the centre of the full strip, with their sticky sides facing. Cut this combined strip into three 7.5 cm (3 in) long pieces.

4 Attach one of these rope holders to the bottom edge of the dispenser with one of its sticky edges, with its remaining exposed sticky edge facing inward. Cut a 30.5 cm (12 in) piece of rope and place it lengthwise across the inner side of one of the holder pieces, across the non-sticky horizontal strip. Fold this holder piece over the rope onto the inner side of the dispenser.

5 Repeat Step 4 with the other two rope holders, spacing each of them 5 cm (2 in) apart. Pull both ends of the rope to close the opening to 5 cm (2 in) in diameter. Tie the ends of the rope in a double knot.

6 Cut six 28 cm (11 in) strips of white duct tape and combine them in pairs, one on top of the other

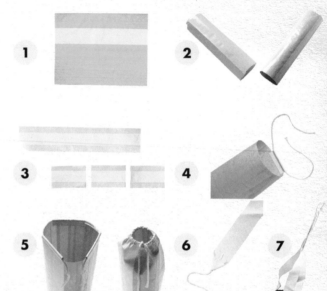

with sticky-sides facing, to create three double-sided strips. Cut the remaining rope into three equal 20.5 cm (8 in) long pieces. Attach one rope to one end of each white strip with glue dots. Wrap each strip's corners around the ropes and secure them with additional pieces of white duct tape.

7 Attach these three strips to the top edge of the bag dispenser with smaller strips of white duct tape, spacing them 5 cm (2 in) apart (as with the rope holder pieces in Step 5). These are the hangers – tie the ends of the ropes together and your dispenser is ready to use.

Materials
» Red duct tape
» White duct tape

16. Table Runner

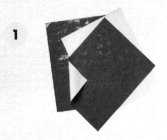

1 Make three double-sided layered fabrics measuring 51 cm (20 in) wide by 40.5 cm (16 in) high. Each should have one red side and one white side. Square up the sides.

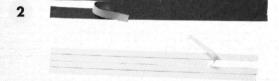

2 Cut one strip of red duct tape and one strip of white duct tape, each measuring 30.5 cm (12 in) long. Working lengthwise, cut smaller 1.25-cm (½-in) high strips.

3 Use the strips of red duct tape to attach the fabric pieces together along the red edges that measure 40.5 cm (16 in) across. Flip the fabrics over and repeat this step using the white duct tape strips. Discard any extra strips. You should now have one single fabric measuring 152 cm (60 in) long.

4 Cut three 51 cm (20 in) lengths of white duct tape. Working lengthwise, cut smaller 1.25 cm (½ in) wide strips. Place the white duct tape strips approximately 1.25 cm (½ in) from the outer edge of the red side. Remove any excess tape.

3   4

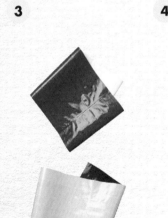

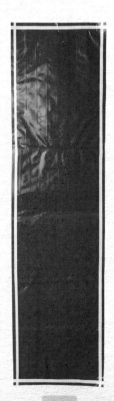

17. Fork and Knife Place Mat

Materials
» White duct tape
» Green duct tape
» Silver chrome duct tape

Additional Tools
» Thin black marker

1 Make a double-sided layered fabric measuring 40.5 cm (16 in) wide by 30.5 cm (12 in) high, white on the front side and green on the back. Square up the sides.

2 Cut three 20.5 cm (8 in) lengths of silver chrome duct tape. On each strip use a thin black marker to draw a fork, a knife, and a spoon. Cut out the shapes with a craft knife, then gently pry them up.

3 Place the knife on the left side, 2.5 cm (1 in) in from the bottom and left edges. Place the fork on the right side, 2.5 cm (1 in) from the bottom and right edges. Place the spoon at the top lengthwise, 2.5 cm (1 in) inward from the top edge and centred.

1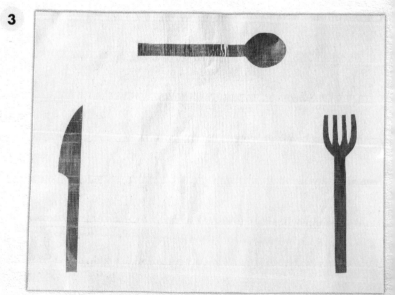

2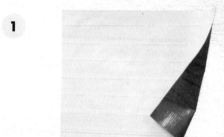

3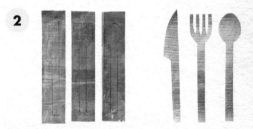

Materials

» Royal blue duct tape
» Black duct tape

Additional Tools

» White grease pencil

18. Vase

1 Make two double-sided layered fabrics 20.5 cm (8 in) wide and 35.5 cm (14 in) high, each with one blue and one black side. Cut a 35.5 cm (14 in) strip of black duct tape and cut it into four 1.25 cm (½-in) wide strips.

2 Attach the two fabric pieces together along their 20.5 cm (8 in) sides with one of the black duct tape strips. Do the same on the opposite, blue side with another strip of black tape. Cut off any excess tape overlapping the fabric's edges.

3 Fold the fabric in half along the seam, with the blue sides facing each other. Orientate the fabric so the folded side is at the bottom edge.

4 Use the remaining strips of black duct tape to close the seams at the left and the right edges. This is the main hollow of the vase.

5 Use one hand to push one of the bottom corners inward, then grab the pushed-in corner with the other hand from the inside of the hollow. Pull the fabric inside-out. Smooth out any wrinkles by hand and then lay it flat on the cutting mat.

6 Cut a 35.5 cm (14 in) strip of royal blue duct tape. Cut it lengthwise into 1.25-cm (½-in) wide strips. Take two strips and cover up the seams on the left and right sides of the vase.

(Continued overleaf)

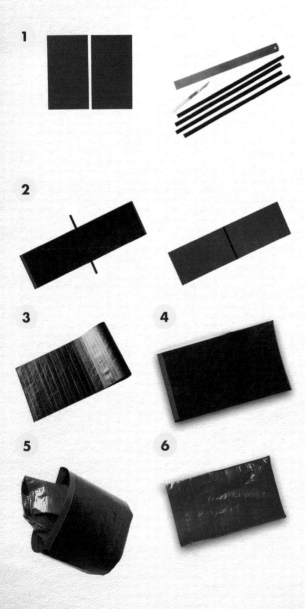

7 From the left corner at the bottom edge, measure and mark 5 cm (2 in) inward toward the centre with the white grease pencil. Pinch the corner to form a triangle. Fold at the 5 cm (2 in) mark, and pull inward toward the centre. Hold this in place with one of the extra pieces of black duct tape.

8 Repeat Step 7 on the right corner.

9 Cover the bottom of the vase with a strip of royal blue duct tape,

19. Duct Tape 'Painting'

1 Make a white, single-sided layered fabric that is 40.5 cm (16 in) wide by 35.5 cm (14 in) high. Use light brown duct tape to make another fabric that is 40.5 cm (16 in) wide and 20.5 cm (8 in) high; then use the craft knife to cut a downward curve into this fabric, from its top right corner toward its bottom left corner, to make a hill shape. Affix this shape to the white fabric, near its bottom edge, and square up the sides. Pry up the white fabric and lay it on the cutting mat with the sticky side facing up. Place the handkerchief on top and smooth out any air bubbles by hand.

2 Cut out branch shapes from the dark brown duct tape. Affix them to the main fabric's white and light brown background, pointing diagonally upward from the bottom right corner.

3 Trace and cut out the crow stencil (see page 49); then make a single-sided layer fabric from black duct tape. Trace the crow shape onto this fabric with a white grease pencil, then cut it out with a craft knife. Cut a small oval shape from a strip of duct tape, in a colour of your choice, to attach as the crow's eye.

4 Gently pry up the crow shape and affix it to the main fabric, filling the white space.

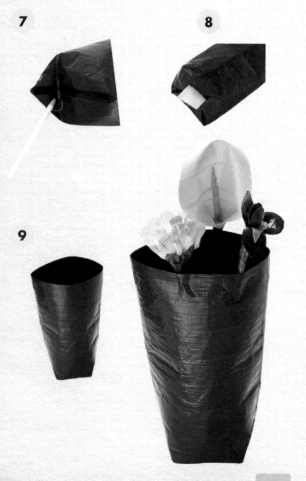

7

8

9

Materials

» White duct tape
» Light brown duct tape
» Dark brown duct tape
» Black duct tape
» Green duct tape
» Crow stencil (see page 49)
» Thin white cotton handkerchief

Additional Tools

» Pencil
» White grease pencil

5 Make a leaf template measuring about 6.25 cm (2½ in) long and 2.5 cm (1 in) wide, and tapering at the base. Trace this template five times onto a 30.5 cm (12 in) strip of green duct tape with a white grease pencil, and cut out the shapes.

6 Gently pry up the leaves and affix them to the upper left corner of the painting.

1

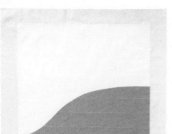

2

3

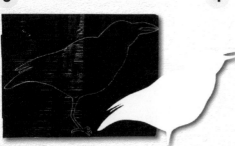

4

5

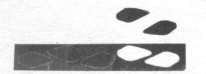

6

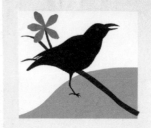

20. Beverage Cozy

Materials

» Silver duct tape
» Black duct tape
» White duct tape
» Bubble insulation
» Velcro® strip, 19 mm (¾ in) wide and 10 cm (4 in) long: side "A" should be 9.5 mm (⅜ in) wide, and side "B" 19 mm (¾ in) wide

1 Cut a rectangular piece of bubble insulation which measures 12.25 cm (5 in) high by 25.5 cm (10 in) wide.

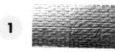

2 Cover one side of the insulation with silver duct tape; lay it lengthwise and with each strip overlapping the other by 3 mm (⅛ in). Extend the duct tape 1.25 cm (½ in) beyond the edge of the insulation.

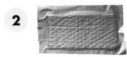

3 Flip the shape over vertically. Use a craft knife and metal ruler to trim the edges of the duct tape fabric to create clean lines. Cut the excess at each of the four corners at a 45-degree angle.

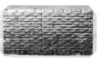
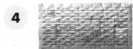

4 Fold the duct tape over the bubble insulation on all four sides, creating tight and clean edges.

5 Affix side "A" of the Velcro® strip vertically along the beverage cozy's right edge. Flip the cozy over horizontally and affix side "B" of the Velcro® strip to the right edge.

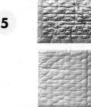
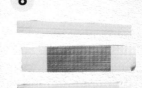

6 Cut a strip of silver duct tape 2.5 cm (1 in) wide and 6.25 cm (2½ in) long. With its sticky side facing up, cover it with a second piece of silver duct tape which extends beyond its top and bottom edges by 2.5 cm (1 in) on each side. Flip this strip vertically so the sticky top and bottom ends are facing upward. Trim off excess sticky parts down the left and right edges.

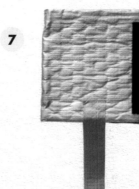
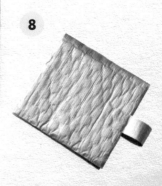

7 Fold the beverage cozy vertically in half. Place the strip, sticky side down, along the centre of the bottom edge.

8 Flip the cozy vertically. Take the other end of the strip and place it, sticky side down, along the centre of the bottom edge. This forms the seat of the beverage cozy.

9 Make a 10.25 cm (4 in) square one-sided layered fabric (see page 8) with black duct tape. Place it on the front of the beverage cozy, 2.5 cm (1 in) from the left edge. With the craft knife, cut out a colon (:) and closed bracket ( )) from a piece of white duct tape. Place these in the centre of the black square, and arrange them to resemble a sideways happy face emoticon (:)).

9

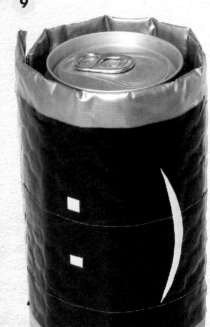

Materials

» Royal blue and white duct tape
» Cork shelf liner, approximately 11.5 cm x 11.5 cm (4½ in x 4½ in)

21. Beverage Coaster

1 Measure the width of one roll of duct tape, double this measurement, and cut two lengths of blue duct tape and two of white. Cut all four of these strips in half lengthwise.

2 Make the woven fabric. To create a checkered design, lay the blue strips down on the mat lengthwise first. Weave the white strips in. You should end up with a perfectly square checkered fabric.

3 Gently pry the fabric up and then lay it down with the sticky side facing upward. Remove the backing from the cork contact paper and place it on top of the duct tape fabric.

4 Flip the coaster over and trim the excess cork to create a cork border around the fabric equal to the width of one square of the pattern.

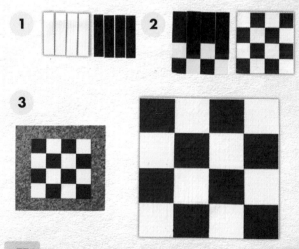

CHAPTER 3:

Cushions, Pads, Mats, and Pillows

Pushing the boundaries of duct tape means looking past its plastic sheen and realizing its potential as a fabric. There is a softer side to duct tape that most people cannot wrap their brains around until they see it—and touch it—for themselves. Perhaps the best example of this is the duct tape pillow.

When I tell people that I make duct tape pillows, I am met with a skeptical look, and the comments that follow are polite and a little condescending—but as soon as I hand them one of my pillows, I know that I have converted another disbeliever.

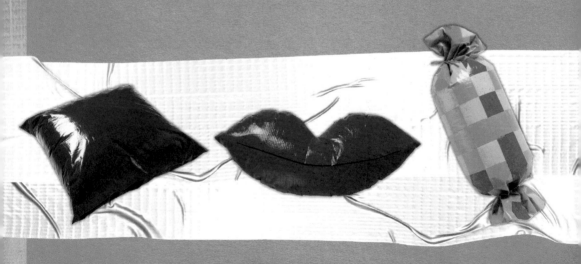

Materials

» Red duct tape
» White duct tape

Additional Tools

» Two pieces of thin cloth (at least 17 in. (43 cm) square (e.g. an old t-shirt/bandana)
» A bag of fiberfill (or any cotton/synthetic stuffing)

22. Seat Cushion

1 Make two striped, one-sided layered fabrics from red and white duct tape, each measuring 17 in. x 17 in. (43 cm x 43 cm). Pry them up and place them on top of the cutting mat sticky-side-up. Lay one of the pieces of cloth over each of their surfaces, smooth out any air bubbles by hand, and trim off any excess.

2 Place one fabric on the cutting mat with the striped side facing up, and the other directly on top with its cloth side facing up. Close up three of the four seams with strips of white duct tape, forming a large pocket. Trim off any excess tape at the corners.

3 Carefully turn the entire pocket inside out. This is the completed cushion cover.

4 Along the bottom edge (opposite the open end), measure 1 in. (2.5 cm) inward from the bottom left and right corners. Pinch the corners, fold them inward at these marks, and hold them in place with small pieces of white tape.

5 Fill the cushion with fiberfill, then close the top seam with a strip of white duct tape, and trim any excess tape at the corners. Then repeat Step 4 in order to create square corners on this seam.

6 To finish off the cushion, wrap a strip of white duct tape lengthwise around all four sides.

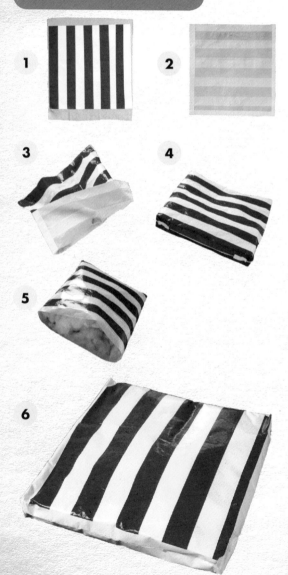

1
2
3
4
5
6

23. Back Pillow

Materials

» Red duct tape
» Leopard print duct tape
» One piece of thin cloth, at least 24½ in. (63 cm) wide by 15 in. (38 cm) high
» Fiberfill

Additional Tools

» Bone folder

1 Make a striped one-sided layered duct tape fabric 23½ in. (59.5 cm) wide by 14 in. (35.5 cm) high. Create stripes in the fabric in whatever arrangement you prefer.

2 Pull up the fabric, lay it on the cutting mat sticky-side-up, and affix a piece of thin cloth over its surface, trimming any excess.

3 Fold the duct tape fabric in half so that its top and bottom sides meet; run the bone folder along the crease to tighten the fold. Cut a 24 in. (61 cm) long strip of red duct tape and cut it in half lengthwise. Use one of these strips to seal the fabric's open seam.

4 Cut the remaining duct tape strip into two 12-in. (30.5-cm) lengths, and use one of these strips to seal one of the pillow's side seams.

5 Stuff the pillow with fiberfill through its open end. Once it reaches the desired firmness, seal the open seam with the remaining strip of red duct tape, and trim any excess duct tape at the corners.

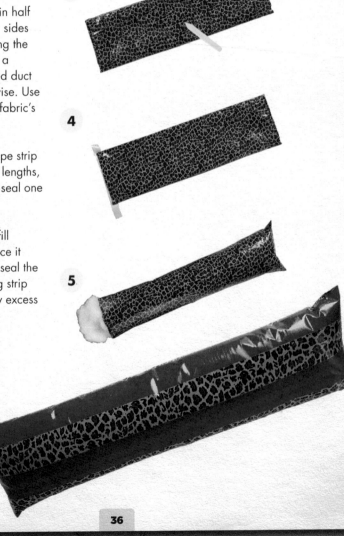

3

4

5

Materials

» Deep ocean blue duct tape
» Black duct tape
» Two pieces of thin cloth,
  each at least 27 in.
  (68.5 cm) square

24. Square Pillow Cover

1 Use deep ocean blue duct tape to make a one-sided layered fabric 25½ in. (65 cm) square. Flip this fabric over and lay it on the cutting mat sticky side facing upward. Roll one of the pieces of thin cloth over the sticky surface and trim any excess cloth from the edges. This is the front panel of the pillow cover. Flip it over again and set it aside.

2 Repeat Step 1 to create a back panel to the same specifications, but using black duct tape. With this back panel's cloth side facing upward, place the front panel directly on top with its cloth-covered side facing downward.

3 Cut two 26-in. (66-cm) long strips of blue duct tape, then cut each strip in half lengthwise. Use three of these strips to seal the seams between the two combined panels on three sides, leaving one side open. Trim off any excess duct tape at the corners.

4 Place a pillow inside the cover through the remaining opening. Use the final strip of blue duct tape to close the open seam.

2

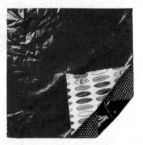

3

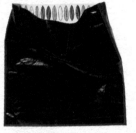

4

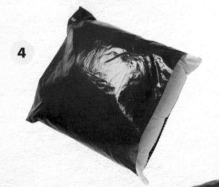

25. Red Heart Pillow

Materials

» Red duct tape
» One sheet of brown paper
» Two pieces of thin cloth, each at least 12 in. (30.5 cm) square
» Bag of fiberfill

Additional Tools

» White grease pencil

1 Fold the brown paper in half and draw half of a heart shape, with the paper's fold as its vertical center. It should measure 12 in. (30.5 cm) high and, when folded, 6 in. (15.25 cm) wide. Cut this stencil out and unfold it.

2 Make two one-sided layered fabrics with red duct tape, both larger than the heart stencil. Trace the stencil onto the fabrics with a white grease pencil, trim the fabrics along these lines, and lay them on the cutting mat sticky-sides-up. These are the pillow's front and back panels.

3 Affix pieces of cloth to the panels' sticky surfaces, and trim any excess cloth from the sides. Then place one fabric directly on top of the other, with their cloth-covered sides facing inward.

4 Cut two 20-in. (52-cm) long strips of red duct tape. Cut a series of "X"-shapes across them, each approximately 2 in. (5 cm) apart, to create hexagonal pieces of tape. Use these to seal the seam between the pillow's two panels; place the hexagons' outer points along the seam, with each tip meeting the next. Leave a 6 in. (15.25 cm) opening unsealed.

5 Stuff the pillow with fiberfill to the desired firmness, and seal the open seam with more hexagonal strips.

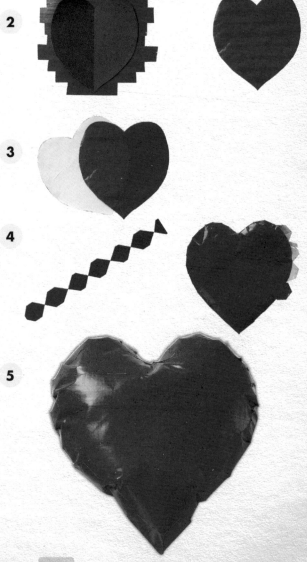

26. Meditation Mat

Materials

» Zebra print duct tape
» Red duct tape
» Black duct tape
» Quilt batting (twin bed size if possible)

Additional Tools

» White grease pencil

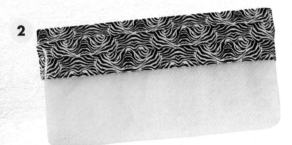

2

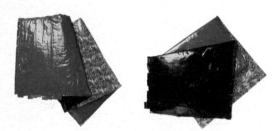

3

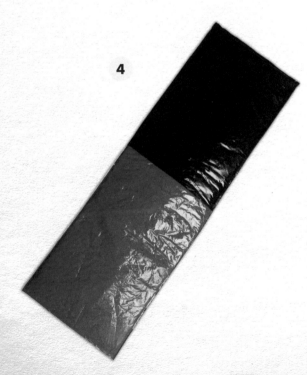

4

1 Fold the quilt batting in half lengthwise. Cut through the two layers of batting (ideally using a rotary cutter if you have access to one, though large scissors will do fine), trimming it down to 2 ft. (61 cm) wide by 6 ft. (183 cm) long.

2 Place the batting on the cutting mat, letting its long end hang over the top edge of the mat and worktable. Starting at the bottom edge of the batting, cover the surface with zebra print duct tape by making a one-sided layered fabric over it. Once you've covered the portion of it that is on top of the cutting mat, lift it up and reposition it to covering the section of batting that is still exposed. Once you reach about halfway up—about 3 ft. (92 cm)—switch to red duct tape.

3 Flip the covered side of the batting over and repeat Step 2 on the exposed side, using red and black duct tapes.

4 Square up the sides neatly, leaving an even trim around the finished mat.

27. Penguin Pillow

Materials

» Black duct tape
» White duct tape
» Orange duct tape
» Two sheets of brown paper
» Two pieces of thin cloth, each at least 22 in. (56 cm) square
» Bag of fiberfill

Additional Tools

» White grease pencil

1 Draw a circle stencil with a 20 in. (51 cm) diameter on brown paper and cut it out.

2 Use black duct tape to make two one-sided layered fabrics, each measuring 22 in. (56 cm) square. Trace the circle stencil on to these fabrics with a white grease pencil, then cut the circle shape out of each fabric with a craft knife.

3 Pry each of the fabrics up and lay them on the cutting mat sticky-side-up. Cover their surfaces with cloth, and trim any excess. Place one fabric directly on top of the other, with their cloth-covered sides facing inward.

4 Cut three 20-in. (61-cm) long strips of black duct tape, and cut a series of "X" shapes across them to create small, roughly hexagonal pieces of tape. Use these to seal the seam between the two panels of the pillow. Place the outer points of the hexagon along the seam, with the tips of each piece slightly overlapping the next. Leave a 6 in. (15.25 cm) opening unsealed.

5 To make a stencil for the penguin's face, first draw and cut out an apple shape, but with elongated sides. It should measure 12½ in. (32 cm) wide by 14½ in. (37 cm) high.

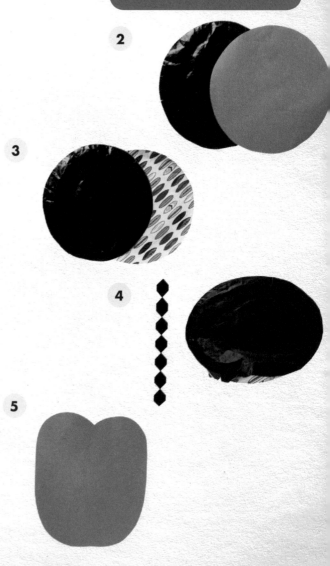

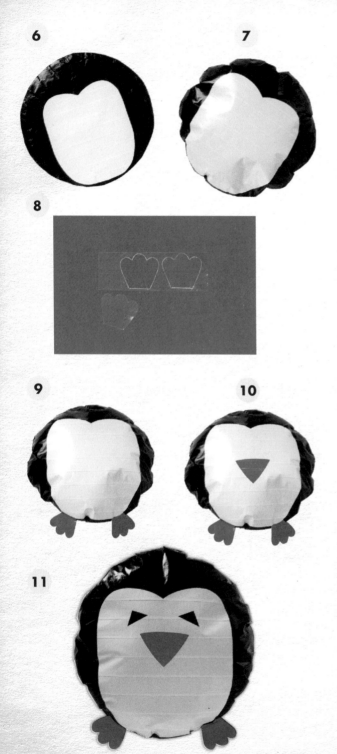

6 Use white duct tape to make a one-sided layered fabric large enough for the stencil to fit inside, then trace the stencils onto the fabric. Cut out this shape and affix it to the front panel of the pillow, centered and almost touching the bottom edge. Keep the opening of the pillow's seam on the left side.

7 Stuff the pillow with fiberfill to the desired firmness, then close the open seam with the remaining hexagonal black duct tape strips.

8 Draw a foot shape onto brown paper and cut it out. Then make a double-sided layered fabric using orange duct tape, 10 in. (25.5 cm) wide and 4 in. (10 cm) high. Trace the foot stencil twice onto the duct tape fabric with a white grease pencil, then cut out the shapes with a craft knife.

9 Affix the heels of the feet to the pillow's bottom edge with thin strips of duct tape, trimmed to match the width of the feet.

10 Trace a triangular beak shape onto brown paper, and cut it out. Make an orange one-sided layered fabric, then trace the stencil on to it and cut it out. Affix the shape to the center of the pillow's front panel, with its apex pointed downward.

11 Cut out a 1½ in. (3.75 cm) square of black duct tape, then halve it diagonally. These are the eyes—affix them above the beak on either side.

28. Travel Diaper Changing Mat

1 Cut three strips of insulation, each 22 in. (56 cm) long and 6 in. (15.25 cm) wide. Lay them on the cutting mat, each of them side by side with no gap between them, in the vertical position.

2 Cover all three strips of insulation with electric blue duct tape by making a single one-sided layered fabric (see page 8).

3 Pry one corner with the craft knife and pull up by hand. Flip over and place it on the mat so the bubble insulation side is facing up. Then cover this side with black duct tape, again making a one-sided layered fabric over it. When this side is sealed, run your fingernail over the seams between each of the insulation strips, which are now covered with black duct tape, so that each of these seams are indented and can act as folding hinges.

4 Square up the sides, leaving a border around the perimeter between ⅛ in. (3.25 mm) and ¼ in. (6.5 mm) wide.

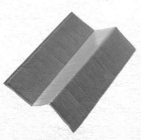

Materials

- » Electric blue duct tape
- » Black duct tape
- » Pipe bubble insulation

29. Red Lips Pillow

1 Create a template for the lips. Fold the brown paper vertically in half, so that it measures at least 14 in. (35.5 cm) square. Draw one side of a pair of lips with a pencil, with its center on the fold. Cut out the shape with scissors through both layers of brown paper, and unfold it. You should have a symmetrical, mouth-shaped template that measures at least 24 in. (61 cm) wide by 12 in. (30.5 cm) high.

2 Make a one-sided layered fabric (see page 8) with red duct tape, approximately 24 in. (61 cm) wide by 12 in. (30.5 cm) high. Place the lips template on top and trace the outline onto the duct tape fabric with black marker. Cut out the lips shape with the craft knife.

3 Gently pull up the duct tape lips and set them aside, sticky side up. Cut off strips of red duct tape approximately 2 in. (5 cm) long. Place them around the outer edges of the lips, halfway overlapping its sides. Start near the bottom center and work around, spacing the strips about ⅛ in. (3.25 mm) apart. As you approach the starting point again, leave an unsealed opening approximately 7 in. (18 cm) wide. Place the thin cotton cloth on top of the fabric's exposed sticky side and press down. Cut off any excess cloth with scissors. Flip the lips over vertically, so that the overlapping tabs are facing upward, and set it aside.

Materials

» Red duct tape
» Black duct tape
» Brown paper
» A piece of thin cloth
» A bag of fiberfill (or any cotton synthetic stuffing)

Additional Tools

» Black marker
» Pencil

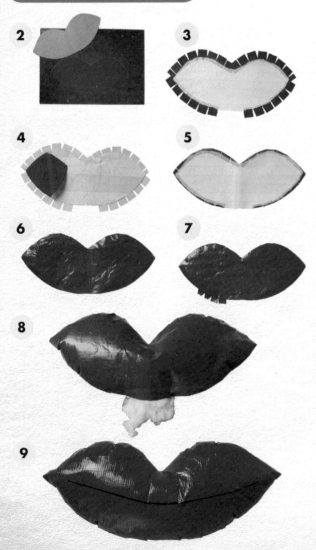

4 Repeat Step 2, creating another red, single sided, lip-shaped duct tape fabric. Pull up this second piece and place it, sticky-side-up, directly on top of the first piece with their edges exactly aligned.

5 Fold the overlapping tabs of the first fabric over onto the second one, fixing both fabrics together and creating as tight a seam as possible. Having done this, cover the remaining exposed sticky side with another piece thin cotton cloth, and again remove any excess cloth with scissors. This completes the main body of the pillowcase, though at the moment it is inside-out.

6 Carefully turn the pillowcase right-side out by pushing the left and right corners inward and pulling both corners gently outward through the 7 in. (18 cm) wide opening in the bottom. You should now have a well-formed, red, lips-shaped pillowcase.

7 Cut strips of red duct tape approximately 1½ in. (3.75 cm) long and attach them to the outer edges of the shape, half overlapping. Cut triangular indentations into each of the overlapping strips and then fold these strips over to seal the outer seam, but leave the 7 in. (18 cm) wide opening unsealed.

8 Stuff the pillowcase with fiberfill through the opening, to the desired thickness. Then seal up the opening with red duct tape.

9 Add a long thin strip of black duct tape across the front of the lips to create a smiling mouth.

30. Duck Pillow

Materials

» Yellow duct tape
» Orange duct tape
» Black duct tape
» One sheet of brown paper
» Two pieces of thin cloth, each at least 22 in. (56 cm) square
» Bag of fiberfill

Additional Tools

» White grease pencil

1 Draw a circle stencil with a 20 in. (51 cm) diameter on brown paper and cut it out. Make two one-sided layered fabrics using yellow duct tape, each measuring at least 22 in. (56 cm) square. Trace the stencil onto the duct tape fabrics with a white grease pencil, and cut out the circles with a craft knife.

2 Pry each of the fabrics up and lay them on the cutting mat sticky-side-up. Cover their surfaces with cloth and trim any excess. Then place one fabric directly on top of the other, with their cloth-covered sides facing inward.

3 Cut three 20-in. (52-cm) long strips of yellow duct tape, and cut a series of "X" shapes across them to create small, roughly hexagonal pieces of tape. Use these to seal the seam between the two panels of the pillow: Place the outer points of the hexagon along the seam, with the tips of each piece slightly overlapping the next. Leave a 6 in. (15.25 cm) opening unsealed.

4 Stuff the pillow with fiberfill to the desired firmness. Close up the open seam with more hexagonal strips.

5 Trace a duckbill shape onto brown paper and cut it out. Make a one-sided layered fabric with orange duct tape large enough to cover the duckbill stencil. Trace the stencil onto the fabric and cut out the shape.

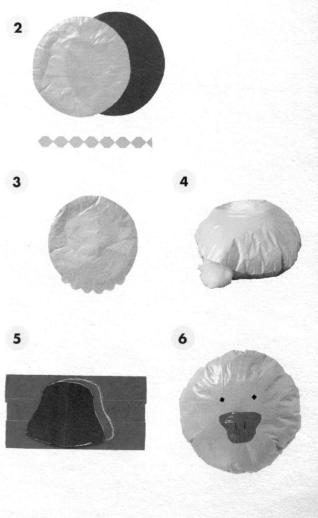

2

3

4

5

6

6 Pull up the duckbill shape and place it on the cutting mat sticky-side-up. Place a small fistful of fiberfill on the duckbill's center, then—keeping the fiberfill in position—affix the bill to the center of the pillow's front panel. Press down around the edges of the duckbill to secure it. Cut two ½ in. (1.25 cm) squares from a small strip of black duct tape. These are the eyes: Pry them up with the craft knife and affix them above the duckbill. Then, from the same strip of black tape, cut two strips 1 in. (2.5 cm) long and ⅛ in. (3.25 mm) wide. Affix these side by side around a third of the way down the duckbill, as the duck's nostrils.

7 Draw a foot shape onto brown paper and cut it out. Then use orange duct tape to make a double-sided layered fabric 10 in. (25.5 cm) wide and 4 in. (10 cm) high; leave a thin sticky border exposed on the reverse side. Trace the foot stencil twice onto the duct tape fabric with a white grease pencil, with the back edge of each foot's heel overlapping onto the sticky border on the reverse. Cut the feet out with a craft knife.

8 Attach the feet to the bottom edge of the pillow using the sticky border on each of their heels, then secure each of them to the pillow with a thin strip of orange duct tape, trimmed to match the width of the feet.

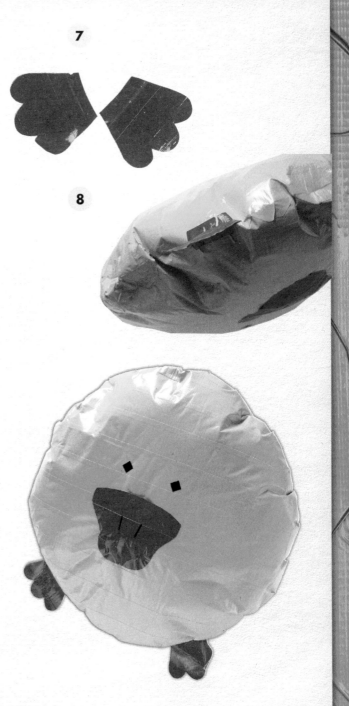

7

8

31. Candy Wrapper Style Pillow

Materials

» Lime green duct tape
» Yellow duct tape
» Hot pink duct tape
» A piece of thin cloth, at least 28 in. (71 cm) wide by 24 in. (61 cm) high.
» Fiberfill

Additional Tools

» Hole puncher, with a diameter of ⅛ to ¼ in. (3.25 to 6.5 mm)
» An awl or pin

1 Make a woven duct tape fabric twelve strips wide by ten strips high, mixing the colors to create a random pattern. Do not square up the sides.

2 Gently pull up the fabric and place it on the cutting mat with its sticky side facing upward. Roll the piece of cloth over the surface, then flip the fabric over and square up the sides.

3 Cut a 24-in. (61-cm) long strip of duct tape of any color, and place it across the cutting mat horizontally, sticky-side-up. Then place the bottom edge of the fabric overlapping halfway over the strip of tape.

4 Fold the fabric's top edge downward so that it meets the bottom edge, forming a cylindrical shape. The overlapping duct tape strip should attach the two ends.

5 Cut a 24-in. (61-cm) long strip of lime green duct tape, and cut a strip measuring ½ in. (1.25 cm) high. Place this strip along the fabric's outside seam.

6 Cut the remaining strip of lime green duct tape in half lengthwise. Twist both strips into two thin ropes.

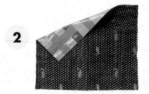
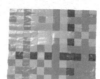

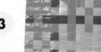

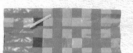

7 At one end of the cover, fold one of the pattern's lengthwise strips over in half, creating a fold. Use the hole-puncher to make a hole through both sides of the fold, 1¾ in. (9.5 cm) inward from the fabric's edge. Repeat this step on each of the other strips around this edge of the fabric, ensuring that the holes are lined up all the way round.

8 Weave one of the thin ropes through the row of holes, using an awl or pin to push the rope through each hole. Pull its ends until the fabric's side is cinched closed, and tie it shut.

9 Stuff fiberfill into the pillow's open end until it reaches the desired size and firmness.

10 Repeat Steps 8 and 9 on the pillow's open end to seal the completed pillow.

6

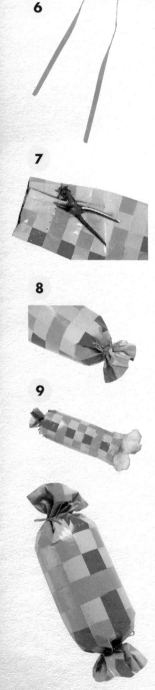

7

8

9

Materials

» Black and white checkered duct tape
» Yellow duct tape
» Silver duct tape
» Parchment paper
» Scrap paper

32. Mouse Pad

1

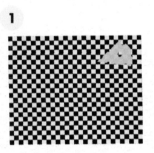

1 Make a double-sided layered duct tape fabric 9½ in. (24 cm) wide by 7½ in. (19 cm) high, one side black-and-white-checkered and the other yellow. Square up the sides. Place a 3-in. (7.5-cm) long strip of yellow tape on a small piece of parchment paper. Cut out a wedge shape, then cut small round holes into it. This is the cheese sticker. Remove the safety backing and affix the sticker to the top-right corner of the checkered fabric.

2

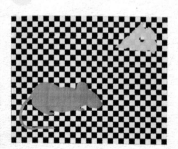

2 Draw a mouse stencil onto brown paper and cut it out. Make a one-sided layered fabric from silver duct tape on top of parchment paper, large enough for the mouse stencil to fit inside. Trace the stencil onto the fabric with a white grease pencil and cut it out. This is the mouse sticker.

3

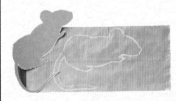

3 Remove the sticker's safety backing and affix it to the bottom-left corner of the checkered fabric to complete your mouse pad.

CHAPTER 4:

Decorative Stickers

I'm sure this experience is not unique to me. I was waiting at the airport's luggage carousel to collect my baggage. After a few minutes I spotted my beat-up black rolling suitcase, and was about to reach for it when a man standing a few feet closer to the action grabbed it. He swiftly rolled away with the receptacle containing a week's worth of my dirty clothes and half-empty bottles of sunblock. I stopped him and pointed out the worn tag with my name on it. He huffed a little, handed me my suitcase, and went back in search of his similar-looking piece of luggage.

So what's the point of my story? A unique sticker would have made all the difference. No suitcase or backpack is unique enough to completely rule out a similar case of mistaken identity—but stick a duct tape peace symbol or butterfly on it and then see if anyone tries to pass yours off as his or her own.

The stickers in this section can not only make that piece of luggage stand out, but can also decorate walls and doors. I've used them to adorn several other projects in this book to give you an idea of how versatile they are. You can even put them on denim jackets or t-shirts. Example stencils are included for you to copy, enlarge, and re-use as many times as you'd like.

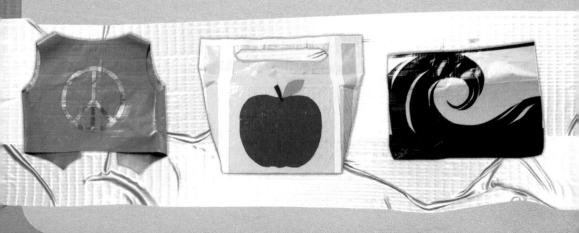

Instructions for All Stencils

1 Create a paper stencil, either by copying, enlarging, and printing the outlines which appear on the following pages, or by drawing it freehand. Set this aside.

2 Make a one-sided layered fabric on top of a sheet of parchment paper, making sure it is large enough for the stencil to fit inside.

3 Place the paper containing the sticker's outline on top of the fabric, and hold it in place with small strips of masking tape at the edges.

4 Cut out the shape with a sharp craft knife. Discard any excess duct tape, masking tape, and parchment paper.

33. Butterfly

34. Crow

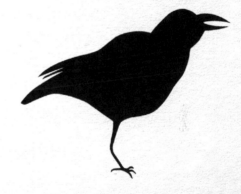

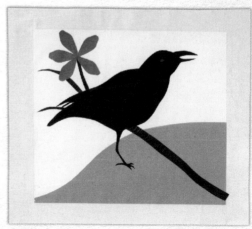

Duct Tape "Painting," page 31

Materials

» Duct tape (in the color or colors of your choice)
» Scrap paper, or a printout of the stencil shape
» Pencil
» Parchment paper

Additional Tools

» Masking tape

35. Red Apple

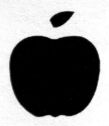

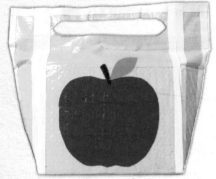

Lunch Bag, page 60

37. Peace Sign

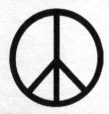

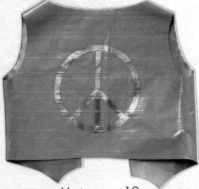

Vest, page 19

36. Sports Car

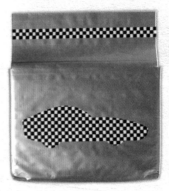

Laptop Case, page 53

38. Sun

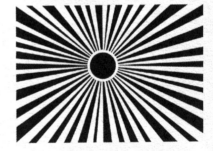

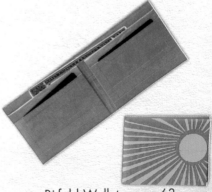

Bi-fold Wallet, page 63

39. Surfing Wave

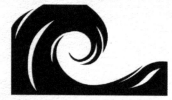

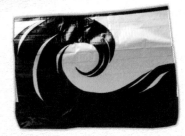

Black and White Clutch, page 54

40. Jolly Roger

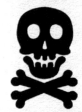

Pirate Hat, page 101

41. Planet Earth

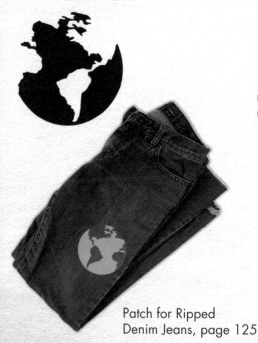

Patch for Ripped
Denim Jeans, page 125

42. Trestle Bridge

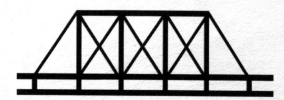

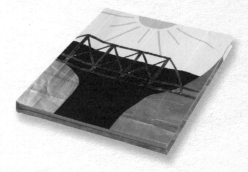

Book Cover, page 124

CHAPTER 5:

Bags, Holders and Wallets

When making any sort of bag, holder or wallet with duct tape you don't have to do one lick of sewing, which makes fixing mistakes or making adjustments a lot easier. Too small? Make an incision and add some more duct tape to it. Too big? Cut it down and then tape it back together. You can add or remove pockets at any time, create a handle where there wasn't one before or transform it completely. That's how accommodating duct tape is as a fabric.

Of course it can become a sticky mess, so it may take a few tries before succeeding. Start with one of the simpler projects in this section, like an ID holder (page 61) or mobile case (page 62). The bigger projects like the beach bag (page 58) are just (much) bigger versions of a mobile case, so the complications won't arise from the instructions so much as from the process of getting used to making and manipulating large duct tape fabrics. The bigger the fabric, the greater the tendency toward clumping, accidental sticking and warping. So start small, master the skills and then attack the bigger projects.

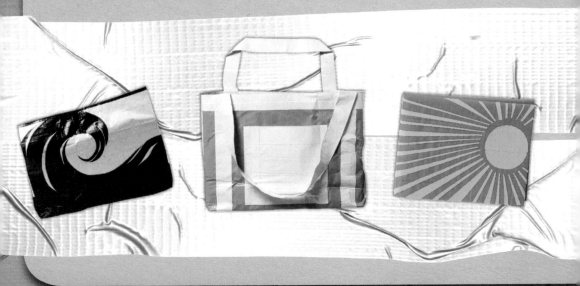

Materials

» Silver duct tape
» Black and white chequered duct tape

43. Laptop Case

1 Make a double-sided layered fabric 35.5 cm (14 in) wide by 12.5 cm (5 in) high, and with one side silver and one chequered. Cut a 40.5 cm (16 in) strip of silver duct tape, then cut it in half lengthwise.

2 Use one strip to attach the two fabrics along their 38-cm (15-in) sides, with their silver sides facing upward. Use the second strip to seal the seam on the opposite side. Fold along this seam so that the two checkered sides face inward.

3 Cut a 30.5 cm (12 in) strip of silver duct tape, then halve it lengthwise. Use these strips to close the left and right seams. This is the main pocket of the case.

4 Mark 1.25 cm (½ in) inward from the bottom-left and -right corners, then pinch both corners and fold them inward along these marks. Hold them in place with small pieces of silver tape, and cover the full length of the bottom edge with a strip of silver tape.

5 Cut an 28 cm (11 in) strip of chequered duct tape, and cut it lengthwise in half. Use these strips to seal the inner side-seams.

6 Use silver and checkered duct tapes to make a double-sided layered fabric measuring 35.5 cm x 12.5 cm (14 in x 5 in).

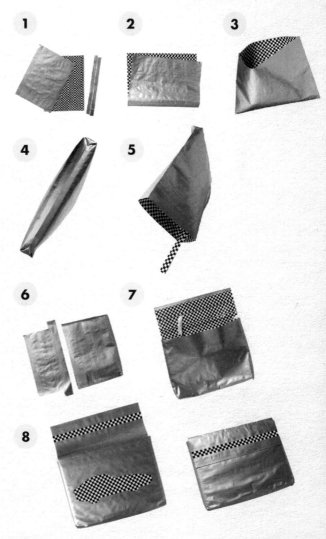

7 Attach the flap to the back of the case with a strip of silver tape, and remove any excess.

8 Cut a 35.5 cm (14 in) strip of chequered duct tape, then cut it in half lengthwise. Use one strip to cover the inside seam between the flap and the case. Affix the other strip across the front flap. To create the Sports Car sticker used above, see page 50.

44. Black and White Clutch Bag

Materials

» Black duct tape
» White duct tape
» One magnetic snap closure (see 'Online Resources', page 128)

1 Make a 30.5 cm x 30.5 cm (12 in x 12 in) double-sided layered fabric, with the top and bottom sections white, and a black section in the middle approximately 12.5–15 cm (5–6 in) high. Square up the sides.

2 Fold the fabric in half so that the centre crease runs lengthwise across the black section in the middle.

3 Cut an 20.5 cm (8 in) strip of black duct tape, and cut it in half lengthwise. Use these strips to seal up the seams on the left and right sides of the folded fabric. Cut off any excess duct tape.

4 Measure inward 2.5 cm (1 in) from the left corner of the bottom seam. Pinch the corner flat to make a triangle, then fold the corner inward along the 2.5 cm (1 in) mark. Hold this in place with a small piece of black duct tape, then repeat this step on the right corner. This will form the main pocket of the clutch bag.

5 Use a 1.25-cm (½-in) wide strip of white duct tape to seal both inside seams.

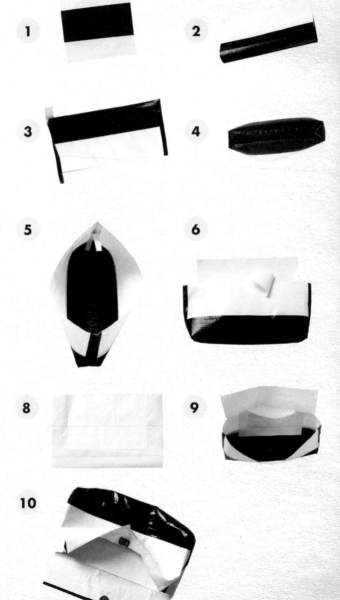

1
2
3
4
5
6
8
9
10

6 Use white duct tape to make a double-sided layered fabric measuring 24 cm (9½ in) wide by 6.25 cm (2½ in) high, and square up its sides. This will form the flap cover – use a strip of white duct tape to attach it to one of the top edges of the clutch bag.

7 Use white duct tape to make two single-sided layered fabrics: one should be 12.5 cm (5 in) wide by 9 cm (3½ in) high, the other 18 cm (7 in) wide by 11.5 cm (4½ in) high. Square up their sides and set the two fabrics aside, sticky-side-up.

8 Place the smaller white duct tape fabric on top of the larger one, aligning the top edges and centring it horizontally.

9 Attach the combined fabrics to the clutch's back inside wall (the one that is attached to the flap cover) to form a pocket.

10 Attach the magnetic snap closure. The 'male' part should be attached to the inside of the cover flap, centred horizontally and approximately 1.25 cm (½ in) from the flap's edge. Cover the metal washer on the top side of the flap with a strip of white duct tape. The 'female' part of the snap closure should be attached to the outside of the clutch bag's front where the flap overhangs. To find the correct position of the female part, attach it to the male part. Close the flap and allow the prongs to make indentations on the opposite clutch bag wall – these indentations will mark where the female part should go. Attach the female part and cover the metal washer with a strip of white duct tape.

For the Surfing Wave sticker used below see page 51.

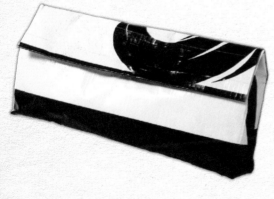

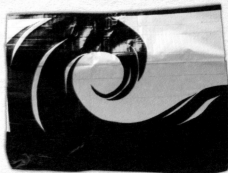

45. Small Tote Bag

1 Use maroon duct tape to make a double-sided layered fabric 30.5 cm (12 in) wide by 23 cm (9 in) high. Square up its sides, then set it aside.

2 Lay the laminating sheet on the cutting mat sticky-side-up. Remove the safety backing and arrange newspaper or magazine clippings on top, with their printed sides facing downward.

3 Cover the back of the laminating sheet with white duct tape, then trim any excess paper or duct tape that falls outside the area of the laminating sheet.

4 Place a strip of white tape across the top edge with its top half overlapping, and fold the strip over onto the opposite side, trimming any excess tape. This is the front panel of the bag.

5 Place the maroon fabric on top of the front panel and line up their edges. Place a strip of white duct tape along the maroon panel's bottom edge, with half of it overlapping. Fold this bottom half onto the front panel.

6 Cut a 23-cm (9-in) long strip of white duct tape and halve it vertically. Place each strip halfway overlapping the sheet's side edges, and fold them over onto the front panel. Trim any excess tape, and carefully turn the pocket inside-out.

Materials

- » Maroon duct tape
- » White duct tape
- » One 23 cm x 30.5 cm (9 in. x 12 in) self-adhesive laminating sheet
- » Newspaper or magazine clippings
- » One 15.25 cm (6 in) strip of Velcro®

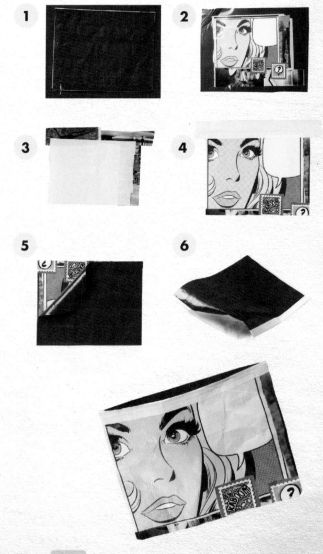

Bags, Holders and Wallets

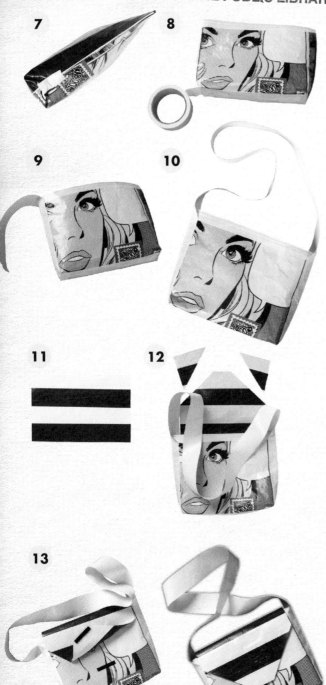

7 On the pocket's back side mark 2.5 cm (1 in) inward from the left and right corners. Pinch both corners and fold them along these marks inward; hold them in place with a small piece of white duct tape.

8 Cover the length of the bottom of the bag with a strip of white duct tape, and use another white strip to secure the inside seam.

9 Cut two 25.5 cm (10 in) strips of white duct tape and affix them to one another, sticky-sides facing. Attach this strip to the top left corner of the bag's main pocket with another white strip running down the length of the bag's left side. Repeat this step on the right side of the bag.

10 Cut a third double-sided strip of white duct tape 40.5 cm (16 in) long and attach it to the loose ends of the two existing strap pieces with white duct tape.

11 Make a striped, double-sided layered fabric 25.5 cm (10 in) wide by 15 cm (6 in) high, using white and maroon duct tape.

12 Attach this fabric to the bag's back panel with a strip of maroon duct tape, so that it acts as a flap. Cut off both of the flap's lower corners at 45-degree angles.

13 Affix side 'A''of the Velcro® tab to the underside of the flap, then attach side 'B' to side 'A' and remove backing from 'B'. Close the flap against the outside of the front panel, ensuring that side 'B' sticks to it.

46. Beach Bag

Materials

» Light blue duct tape
» White duct tape

1 Make a double-sided layered fabric 86.5 cm (34 in) wide by 68.5 cm (27 in) high, with two strips of white on both edges, and the rest light blue. Fold the fabric vertically in half and square up the three open sides.

2 Place white duct tape strips on the fabric's left and right sides, with the outer halves of the tape strips overlapping the edges. Fold the strips over to seal the seams, then trim any excess tape.

3 Carefully turn the pocket inside-out, then repeat Step 2 to seal the exposed seams.

4 Fold the left and right corners over and inward by 10 cm (4 in) along the bottom edge of the bag, and hold these in place with small pieces of duct tape.

5 Mark 3.75 cm (1½ in) inward from the right edge at the top and bottom of the bag. Affix a strip of white duct tape extending from the bag's bottom up its side, with the strip's outer edge aligned with the marks. Extend the strip 30.5 cm (12 in) beyond the bag's top edge – this will form one of the handles.

6 Place a strip of white duct tape over the exposed sticky side of the handle, extending downwards beyond it by at least 25.5 cm (10 in) onto the inside of the bag.

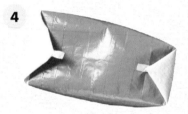
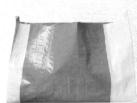
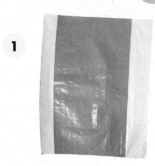

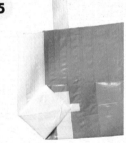

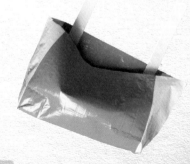

8

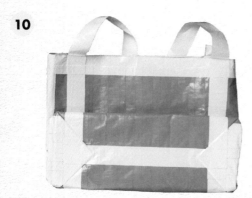

10

11

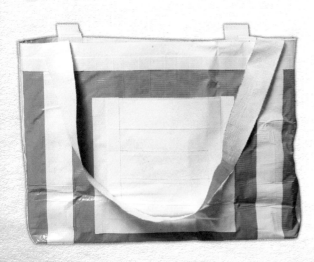

7 Repeat Steps 5 and 6 for the left side of the bag. Attach two equal handle pieces on the opposite side of the bag.

8 To create a seam round the top edge of the bag, first place a strip of white duct tape along this edge, with the top half of the strip overlapping. Then cut another strip of white tape and place it directly on top of the first, from the inside of the bag. Repeat this step on the other side of the main pocket, ensuring that the left and right sides are connected at either end.

9 To finish the handles, mark 2.5 cm (1 in) downward from the loose ends of each of the four handle strips. Cut a 35.5 cm (12 in) strip of white duct tape and use it to attach the two handle strips which extend from the front of the bag, with the end of the new strip aligned with the open strips' 2.5 cm (1 in) marks. Use another 35.5 cm (12 in) strip of white duct tape to cover the sticky side of this handle. Repeat this step to complete the second handle.

10 Place a strip of white duct tape along the bottom seam for extra support.

11 Make a white double-sided layered fabric measuring 20.5 cm x 20.5 cm (8 in. x 8 in). Place strips of white duct tape along three of its sides, and trim them to create an even, 2.5 cm (1 in) sticky border. This is the outside pocket – affix it to the front of the main bag.

47. Lunch Bag

1 Cut the pipe insulation into five pieces: two front and back panels measuring 20.5 cm (8 in) wide by 15 cm (6 in) high, two side panels measuring 10 cm (4 in) wide by 15 cm (6 in) high and a bottom panel measuring 20.5 cm (8 in) wide by 10 cm (4 in) high.

2 Use yellow duct tape to attach the front, bottom and back panels to each other along their 20.5 cm (8 in) edges, with the bottom piece in the middle, and each edge almost – but not quite – touching. Attach the two side panels to either open side of the bottom panel in the same way.

3 Flip the shape over and cover the surface of the upper, back and bottom panels with yellow duct tape, trimming any excess.

4 Cover the right side panel with three strips of duct tape (yellow–white–yellow). Extend the duct tape fabric beyond the panel's edge by 10.25 cm (4 in) so it measures a total of 25.5 cm (10 in). Flip over and cover the sticky side with yellow duct tape. Square up the sides.

5 Add three horizontal yellow duct tape strips extending from the front panel's top edge, with each strip overlapping the others by 1.5 mm (¹⁄₁₆ in). The front panel should now measure 25.5 cm (10 in) in height. Flip over and cover the sticky side with yellow duct tape. Square up the sides.

Materials

» Bubble insulation
» Yellow duct tape
» White duct tape
» Piece of scrap paper at least 18 cm (7 in) wide and 5 cm (2 in) high
» Two Velcro® tabs, each 7.5 cm (3 in) long

Additional Tools

» Pencil

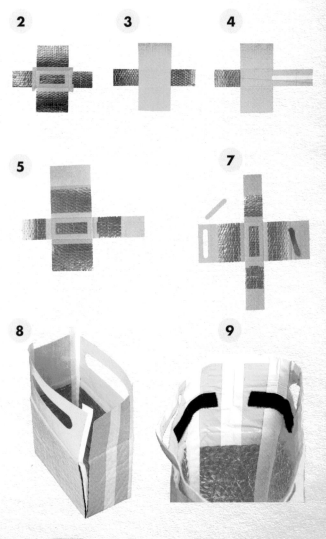

6 Repeat Step 4 on the left panel, and Step 5 on the back panel.

7 Cut out a handle template from scrap paper. It should have rounded sides and measure 15 cm (6 in) wide and 2.5 cm (1 in) high. Position the top edge of the template 2.5 cm (1 in) from the top edge of the front panel, centring it. Trace and cut out the outline of the template, then do the same on the back panel.

8 Cut four 26.5-cm (10½-in) long strips of white duct tape, and halve each of them lengthwise. Use these strips to connect the inner edges of the front, back, left and right panels, then seal the outer edges.

9 Open the lunch bag and affix the two Velcro® tabs horizontally below the handle holes on the bag's left and right sides. Remove the backing from the inner sides of the Velcro® tabs, then close the bag. Firmly press the front and back panels together, then gently open the bag so the Velcro® tabs come apart. The bag should close flat at the top but retain its rectangular shape at its base.

To create the Red Apple sticker used below, see the instructions on page 50.

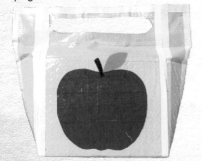

Materials

» Camouflage duct tape
» Transparent duct tape

48. ID Holder

1 Using the camouflage duct tape, make a double-sided layer fabric measuring 6.5 cm x 9 cm (2½ in x 3½ in). Be sure to square up the sides.

2 Using the transparent duct tape, make a double-sided layer fabric measuring 6.5 cm x 9 cm (2½ in x 3½ in). Be sure to square up the sides. Cut out a thumb notch, approximately 1.9 cm (¾ in) wide and 3.25 mm (⅛ in) tall, from the centre of one of the 6.5 cm (2½ in) edges.

3 Cut a 7.5 cm (3 in) strip of transparent duct tape, then cut this lengthwise into 1.25-cm (½-in) wide strips.

4 Place the two fabric pieces on top of each other. Use the transparent tape strips to close up the seams on three sides, leaving the edge with the thumb notch open.

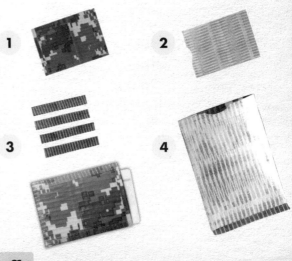

49. Mobile Phone Case

Materials

» Pink and white polka
  dot duct tape
» White duct tape

1 Make a double-sided layer fabric measuring 15 cm (6 in) wide by 11.5 cm (4½ in) high. Be sure to square up the sides. The front side should be all white, but with a 1.25 cm (½ in) pink and white polka dot border along the top edge. The reverse side should be all pink and white polka dot.

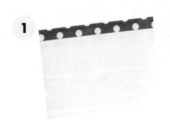

2 Cut a 12.5 cm (5 in) strip of white duct tape, and cut it in half lengthwise. Place one strip overlapping halfway onto the left edge of the fabric.

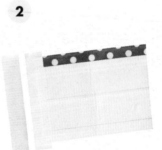

3 Fold the fabric in half vertically so the right edge meets the left edge. Fold the strip of white duct tape over to close the seam, then take the second strip and cover the seam from the inside.

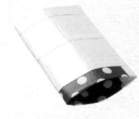

4 Open up the fabric like a loop and then press down on it so the closed seam is vertically in the middle of the bottom layer. This completes the main body of the case.

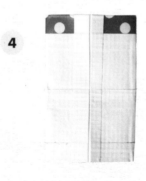

5 Cut a 7.5 cm (3 in) strip of pink and white polka dot duct tape, then cut it in half lengthwise. Take one strip and place it along the bottom edge of the case, overlapping halfway over the edge. Fold it over and close the seam to complete the case.

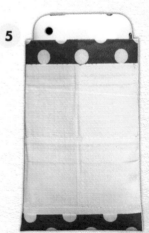

Materials

» Teal duct tape

50. Bi-fold Wallet

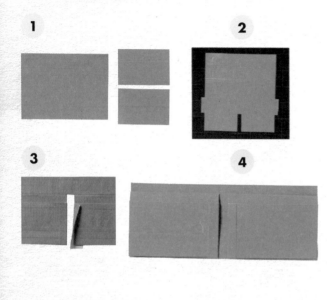

1 Make three double-sided teal layer fabrics, one of them 23 cm (9 in) wide by 16.5 cm (6½ in) high, the other two 11 cm (4¼ in) wide by 7.5 cm (3 in) high.

2 Place the two smaller pieces directly beneath the bottom edge of the large one, with a 1.25 cm (½ in) horizontal gap between them. Use teal duct tape to attach the three pieces.

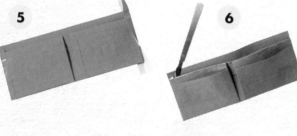

3 Make two double-sided layer fabric pieces measuring 11 cm (4¼ in) wide by 6.5 cm (2½ in) high. Place these two pieces on top of the two smaller pieces now attached to the large fabric, aligning their bottom edges. Use teal duct tape to seal both pockets' inside seams.

4 Fold the pockets back and under the main fabric piece. Mark 9 cm (3½ in) down the large fabric's sides and fold it upward at this mark.

5 Cut a 25.5 cm (10 in) strip of duct tape, and halve it lengthwise. Cut one half into two 12.5 cm (5 in) strips, and use these to seal the wallet's sides.

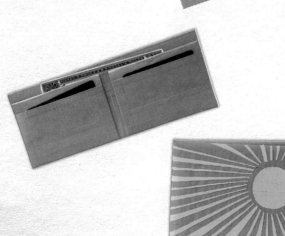

6 Use another 25.5 cm (10 in) strip to seal the bottom seam. Use a craft knife to cut open any mistakenly sealed pockets.

See page 50 for the Sun sticker used to decorate this project.

51. Tri-fold Wallet

Materials

» Black duct tape
» Leopard print duct tape
» 15.25 cm (6 in) strip of Velcro®

1 Make a double-sided layer fabric measuring 20.5 cm (10 in) wide by 17.5 cm (7 in) high. The front side should have a 2.5 cm (1 in) border of leopard print along the top and bottom edges, with the middle a solid black; the reverse side should be all leopard print. Square up the sides. This is the outer part of the wallet.

2 Make a second double-sided layer fabric from black duct tape, measuring 23 cm (9 in) wide by 17.5 cm (7 in) high. Cut this into three equal pieces, each measuring 7.5 cm (3 in) wide by 17.5 cm (7 in) high. These will form the inside pockets.

3 With the outer part of the wallet in the landscape position, lay two of the three inside pockets on top, one on each edge. Cut an 20.5 cm (8 in) strip of black duct tape, then halve it lengthwise. With these two strips, seal the outer seams between the left and right pockets and the wallet's front, outer side.

4 Make two black double-sided layer fabric pieces 8.5 cm (3⅜ in) wide by 3.75 cm (1½ in) high. These will form the card-holders.

5 Take the one remaining 7.5 cm x 17.5 cm (3 in x 7 in) fabric piece and orientate it on the cutting mat in the portrait position. Lay the card-holders end-to-end on top of the large fabric piece, with the right edges of all three pieces aligned. Leave a 6.5 mm (¼ in) gap between the two card holders.

1
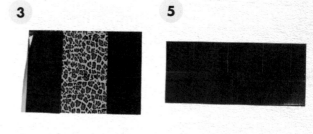

2
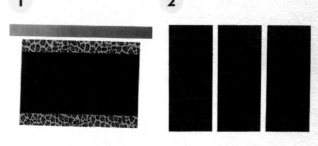

3 **5**
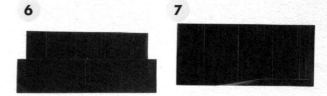

6 **7**

8 **9**
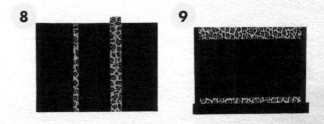

6 Cut an 20.5 cm (8 in) strip of black duct tape and place it over the card holders. Run a fingernail into the space between the holders to tighten the seal.

7 Flip the wallet over. Fold over the extra duct tape so that the card holders are now attached. This is the middle pocket.

8 Place the middle pocket on the wallet, centred between the other two pockets. Cut an 20.5 cm (8 in) strip of leopard print duct tape, and cut it in half lengthwise. Place one of these two strips along the closed edge of the card holders, with a 1.25 cm (½ in) edge overlapping. Fold this edge over onto the wallet, and cut off any excess duct tape.

9 Cut a 26.5 cm (10½ in) strip of black duct tape, then cut it in half lengthwise. Flip over the outer wallet from left to right. Place one of the strips of black duct tape halfway overlapping the bottom edge.

10 Flip the wallet over again from left to right. Cut off the corners of the black strip of duct tape at a 45-degree angle with the craft knife; the centre of the cut should almost touch the corner of the wallet. Fold over the duct tape to seal the seam.

11 Repeat Step 10 for the top edge of the wallet.

12 Use the craft knife to gently cut open any of the pockets that may have been sealed.

13 Add the Velcro® strip to the inner seam of the right inside pocket to seal it. Fold the finished wallet into thirds.

10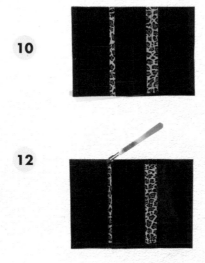

12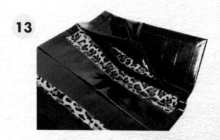

13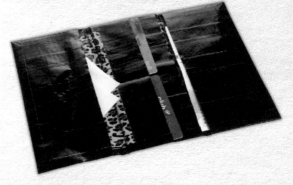

52. Pencil Case

Materials

» Royal blue duct tape
» Transparent duct tape
» 23 cm (9 in) strip of Velcro®

1 Make two 25.5 cm x 12.5 cm (10 in x 5 in) double-sided layer fabrics – one from royal blue and one from transparent duct tapes.

2 Make a third, smaller royal blue double-sided layer fabric. It should measure 25.5 cm x 10 cm (10 in x 4 in).

3 Attach the two blue fabrics along their long sides with a strip of transparent duct tape, then fold them along the seam. Keep the smaller fabric facing upward, as it will form the inner pocket.

4 Place the transparent fabric on top of the combined blue fabrics, aligning their edges. Cut an 28-cm (11-in) long strip of transparent duct tape, and cut it in half lengthwise. Place one strip halfway overlapping along the bottom edge. Cut the excess tape at the corners at 45-degree angles, and fold the tape over to seal the bottom seam.

5 Cut another transparent duct tape strip in half to make two 14 cm (5½ in) lengths. Place each one halfway overlapping each side edge. Cut off each strip's bottom corner at a 45-degree angle, and fold the tape over to close the seams.

6 Affix the Velcro® strip to the inside top edges of the finished pencil case.

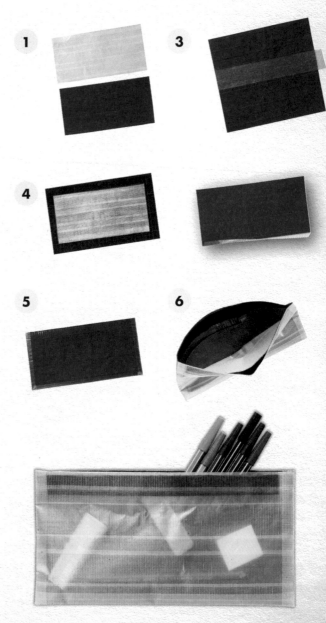

Materials

» 7 in. x 8 in. (18 cm x 20.5 cm) piece of velour or other soft fabric
» Hot rod duct tape

53. Eyeglass Case

1 Make a single-sided layer duct tape fabric measuring 23 cm (9 in) wide by 20.5 cm (8 in). Do not square up the sides.

2 Pull up the fabric by hand in a diagonal motion, and lay it on the cutting mat with the sticky side facing up. Place the velour on top and smooth out any air bubbles. Square up the top, left and bottom sides so there is an exposed sticky 1.25 cm (½ in) border surrounding the velour lining.

3 On the left 20.5 cm (8 in) side, cut halfway slits at a 45-degree angle down- and outward from the top and bottom corners. Fold the resulting trimmed flap of duct tape over onto the inner lining.

4 Cut off the remaining pieces of duct tape at the top and bottom so that the left edge is vertically straight. Then square up the top edge, removing the sticky border.

5 Fold in half by bringing the top edge down to meet the bottom edge. The edges of the velour lining should line-up, leaving the sticky border open. Fold over the sticky border at the bottom, closing the seam.

6 Press down along the right edge to seal it. Use the metal ruler and craft knife to clean up the edge.

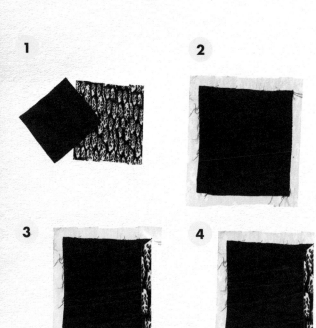

1

2

3

4

5

6

54. Activity Bag

Materials

» White duct tape
» Red duct tape
» Two 15 cm (6 in)
   Velcro® strips

Additional Tools

» Bone folder

1 Make a double-sided layered duct tape fabric measuring 42 cm (16½ in) wide by 54.5 cm (21½ in) high, with the front side red and the reverse side white.

2 With the red side facing upward, pull the bottom edge upward so that its edge sits 6.5 cm (2½ in) below the top edge. Use a bone folder to sharpen the bottom crease.

3 Cut a 23-cm (9-in) long strip of red duct tape, then halve it lengthwise. Place one strip down the bag's left seam, half-overlapping it, and fold the strip over to close the seam. Use the other strip to seal the right seam.

4 Use white duct tape to make a one-sided layered fabric four strips high and 48.5 cm (19 in) wide. Set it aside on the cutting mat with the sticky side facing up. Make a red one-sided layered fabric four strips high and 30.5 cm (12 in) wide. Attach it to the top of the white duct tape fabric along the top edge so that it overlaps by 6.5 mm (¼ in).

5 Along the top edge of the white duct tape fold the red duct tape down, leaving a thin sticky edge exposed beyond the red fabric's edge. This is the outer pocket.

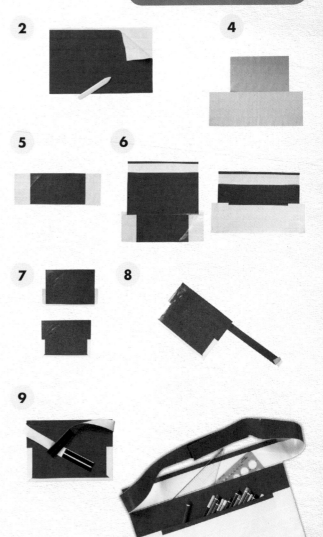

2

4

5

6

7

8

9

6 Rotate the outer pocket by 180 degrees. Place the bottom edge of the front of the bag next to the outer pocket's top edge, making sure it is centred. Attach it with a thin strip of white duct tape, and cut off any excess tape. Fold the outer pocket upward, affixing it to the front of the bag.

7 Flip over so the bag's reverse side is facing upward. Cut off the bottom left and right corners of the sticky overlapping portion of the outer pocket at 45-degree angles. Fold the remaining flaps over the sides.

8 Attach a strip of white duct tape to the left side of the bag, extending 40.5 cm (16 in) horizontally outward from 1.25 cm (½ in) below the bag's top edge. Place a strip of red duct tape over the sticky side of this white strip, overlapping the red strip onto the edge of the bag.

9 Repeat Step 8 on the right side of the bag. Then attach the Velcro® strips to the two ends of the straps to fasten them together. The bag can now be hung over the back of a stroller or the front seat of a car, and filled with books, small toys, games, stationery or whatever you need to keep in it.

Materials

» Black duct tape
» Green duct tape
» White duct tape
» Silver duct tape
» Two 23 cm (9 in) Velcro® strips

Additional Tools

» Magnetic snap closure
» Bone folder

55. Messenger T-Bag

1 Make a woven fabric eighteen strips wide and eleven strips high. Start with the eleven strips running across the width of the cutting mat. Make the fourth horizontal strip from the top white, and all other strips black.

2 Place three rolls of duct tape along the top edge, starting from the top-left corner, in order to measure the width of three strips. Lift and fold over the ends of the following horizontal duct tape strips, starting from the top: 1, 2, 6, 7, 8 and 10 (leave the others stuck down). Affix a vertical white duct tape strip running downward across the stuck-down strips, beginning immediately to the right of the three duct tape rolls. Replace the lifted black duct tape strips on top of the white strip.

2

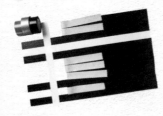
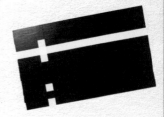

3 To the immediate left of the white vertical strip, weave in a green duct tape strip. Start with the top horizontal strip in the down position. Then continue to weave in two more green strips to the left of the first, but leave the horizontal white strip up until the weave is complete.

4 Weave fourteen vertical green strips to the right of the vertical white strip to complete the woven fabric, again starting with the top horizontal strip in the up position.

5 Carefully pry the fabric up off the cutting mat, flip it over from top to bottom, and lay it down sticky-side-up. Cover this sticky side with a silver, one-sided duct tape fabric. Square up the sides.

6 Flip the fabric over from top to bottom. Measure six vertical strips inward from the right edge, then fold the right edge over at this mark and reinforce the crease with a bone folder. Rotate the fabric 90-degrees clockwise so the crease now runs along the bottom edge. This is the bag's main pocket.

7 Cut a 26.5 cm (10½ in) strip of silver duct tape, then cut it in half lengthwise. Open the left side of the bag and place one of the silver strips halfway overlapping the edge of the back seam. Fold the strip in half so that it is flush with the left edge, and use the strip's exposed sticky side to close the left seam of the bag. Repeat this step on the right side.

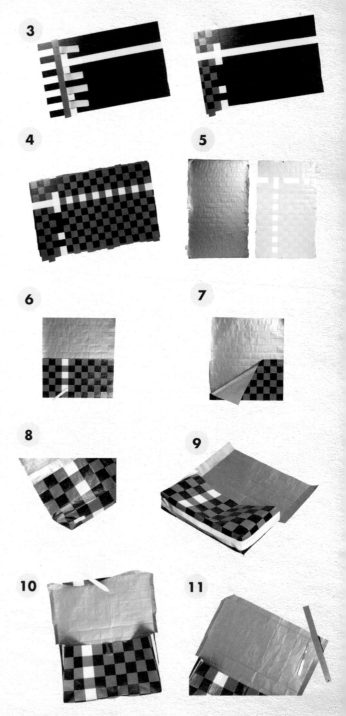

8 On the bottom seam, measure and mark 5 cm (2 in) inward from the left and right corners. Pinch each corner to make a triangle, then fold them inward along the marks. Secure them with small pieces of white tape.

9 Affix a single strip of white duct tape down the centre of one outer side-seam, along the bottom seam and back up the opposite side seam. Fold over any excess at either top edge.

10 At the point where the top of the pocket meets the open flap, make a horizontal cut inward from the left and right sides, measuring the width of one strip, to create two flaps. Fold these flaps inward. Then mark 2.5 cm (1 in) from the top edge of the flap and fold it horizontally along this mark. Use a bone folder to tighten all three creases, then unfold them.

11 Cut the top left and right corners off at 45-degree angles, with the cuts bisecting the perpendicular points where the vertical and horizontal folds meet. Fold the edges over and secure them in place with silver duct tape on the inside of the flap.

12 The bag's flap should have a turnover one strip wide. To add straps, affix two lengths of silver duct tape to the inside of this turnover, and extend them 61 cm (24 in) outward beyond the edges of the bag. Cover these strips' sticky sides with strips of black duct tape, overlapping the black strips over onto the top side of the turnover. Cover the straps' silver sides again with strips of green tape. Then attach the Velcro® strips to the two ends of the straps to fasten them together.

13 To add the magnetic snap closure, first attach the 'male' part of the closure to the inside of the front flap, positioning it in the centre approximately 2.5 cm (1 in) from the bottom edge. Cover the metal washer on the top side of the flap with a small strip of black duct tape. Then, to find the correct position of the 'female' part, attach it to the male part and close the flap, allowing the prongs to make indentations on the outer surface of the bag's pocket. Attach the clasp's female part to the bag where indicated by these indentations, and cover the metal washer on the bag's inner side with a piece of silver duct tape.

12

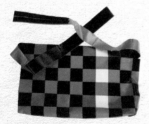

13

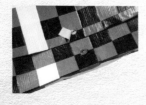

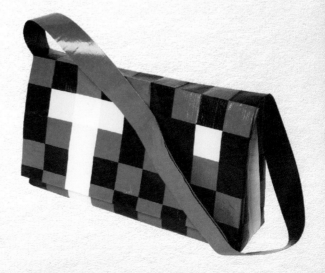

CHAPTER 6:

Flowers

It seems counterintuitive to love shiny fake flowers, particularly if you have an actual garden full of real blooming beauties. But the appeal of these faux florals is undeniable. Anyone who encounters a duct tape rose will find themselves smiling and nodding his or her head at the clever use of such an industrial material.

These projects look harder to make than they really are – the basic technique of rolling the strip loosely in one hand is not an original one, as you may recognize from having made paper flowers. It's easy once you get the hang of it, and making a dozen duct tape tulips for your dining table centrepiece can be done quite quickly. Heck, it might even be faster than running to the closest flower shop for the real ones – as well as a lot more fun and satisfying!

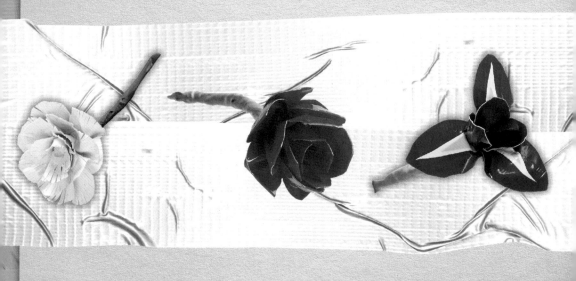

Materials

» White duct tape
» Yellow duct tape
» Green duct tape
» Scrap paper for template

56. Calla Lily

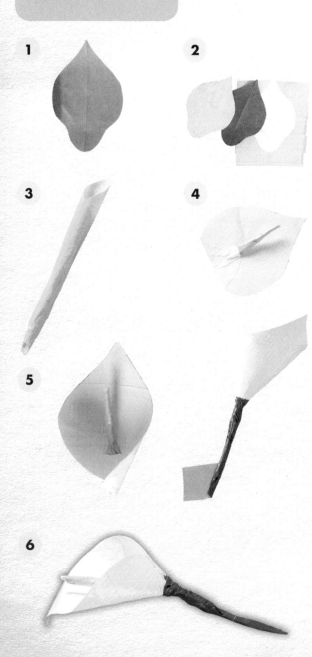

1 Draw and cut out a petal stencil 19 cm (7½ in) high and 13.5 cm (5¼ in) across at its widest point.

2 Then make a double-sided layered fabric with white duct tape, 16.5 cm (6½ in) wide by 19 cm (7½ in) high; leave a 1.25-cm (½-in) high strip of the sticky side exposed. Align the fabric's sticky strip with the stencil's bottom edge, trace the stencil's outline onto the fabric and cut it out.

3 Cut a 15.25 cm (6 in) strip of yellow duct tape. From one of its corners roll the length of the strip at a slight diagonal angle so the end tapers into a point, and the finished shape is 10 cm (4 in) long. This is the flower's pistil.

4 Place the pistil on the centre of the white petal, with the points of both shapes aligned; the pistil's bottom edge should touch the top edge of the sticky strip. Fold the sticky strip forward over the base of the pistil, and press down to secure it.

5 Pull the lower sides of the flower inward, making it cone-shaped. Cut a 30.5-cm (12-in) long strip of green duct tape, and wrap it tightly around the petal's base, securing the cone shape. After two revolutions, twist the strip downward to form the stem.

6 Pull the tip of the flower backward.

57. Red Rose

Materials

» Red duct tape
» Green duct tape

1 Cut a strip of red duct tape measuring 30.5 cm (12 in) long, then flip it over so the sticky side is facing up. Just as you would begin to make a double-sided layer fabric, fold the strip lengthwise so that only a 6.5 mm (¼ in) strip of the sticky side remains.

2 With the sticky side facing inward, begin to wind the strip in a spiral.

3 As you wind the strip, pinch the sticky end, and allow some space between the layers.

4 When you are done winding, give the sticky end a few tight pinches to ensure that it won't come apart. This completes the basic shape of the flower. Set this aside.

5 Cut a strip of green duct tape measuring 20.5 cm (8 in) long. Starting from the right side cut 'V'-shaped pieces out of the top edge until you reach approximately 7.5 cm (3 in) inward.

6 Pry the right side up with the craft knife, and pull the strip up by hand. Starting with the upper right edge, place the green strip along the bottom of the rose. Separate the peaks between the 'V' cuts. Tightly pinch together the bottom edge of the strip as you roll it around the rose.

7 Once you make it one time around the rose, twist the green strip into a stem.

8 Use the detail scissors to cut out the rose petals, which should be shaped like thumbs. Be sure to round the corners. Fluff out the petals when you are done.

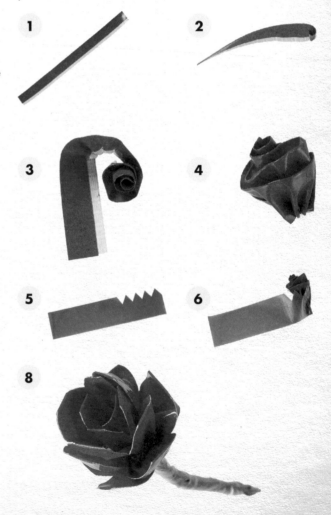

1
2
3
4
5
6
8

Materials

» Yellow duct tape
» Maroon duct tape
» Lime green duct tape
» Fibrefill

Additional Tools

» Thin black marker

58. Sunflower

1 Cut four 16.5 cm (6½ in) strips of maroon duct tape, pair them up and overlap their horizontal edges by 3.25 mm (⅛ in) to create two rectangles.

2 Place a small fistful of fibrefill on the sticky centre of the back panel, affix the front panel directly on top and press down the edges. Trace a circle around the stuffing using the inside of a duct tape roll, then cut it out.

3 Begin to make a double-sided layered fabric 51 cm (20 in) wide from yellow duct tape, but stop when its height reaches 7.5 cm (3 in), and keep the sticky side unfinished facing down. Place strips along the fabric's top and bottom edges to hold it in place.

4 Draw and cut out at least twenty petals 1.25 cm (½ in) wide and 7.5 cm (3 in) long, with pointed tips; their bottoms should be square, and sticky on one edge.

5 Attach each petal to the back of the flower's centre; begin with the 12, 3, 6 and 9 o'clock positions to ensure symmetry.

6 Cut two 16.5 cm (6 in) strips of lime green duct tape, and overlap their horizontal edges by 3 mm (⅛ in). Use the inside of the duct tape roll to trace a circle around the centre, and cut out this circle. Pry it up and then affix it to the back of the sunflower.

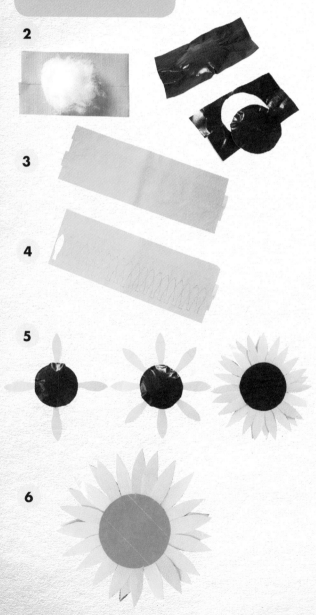

2

3

4

5

6

59. Cherry Blossom Branch

Materials

» Pink and white polka dot duct tape
» Maroon duct tape
» Brown duct tape
» 24-gauge steel wire, at least 40.5 cm (16 in) long
» Mini glue dots

1 Cut a 15.25-cm (6-in) long strip of pink and white polka dot duct tape. With its sticky side facing upward, fold the strip over lengthwise so that only a 6.5 mm (¼ in) strip of the sticky side remains exposed.

2 Use a craft knife to cut five slits into the strip extending downward to slightly above the sticky strip, creating six 2.5 cm (1 in) wide sections. These six sections will become the petals.

3 Fold one petal inward so that its left and right sides meet, with its sticky side facing outward. Then fold its outer edges back toward the middle, creating an accordion fold. Pinch its base to make this fold permanent. Repeat this on the other five petals.

4 Connect the strip's first and last petals at the base with a glue dot to create a circular blossom. On the back of the shape, give the centre a tight pinch to ensure that the petals stick together.

5 Use detail scissors to round each petal's corners.

6 Repeat Steps 1 to 5 three times more, until you have four blossoms in total.

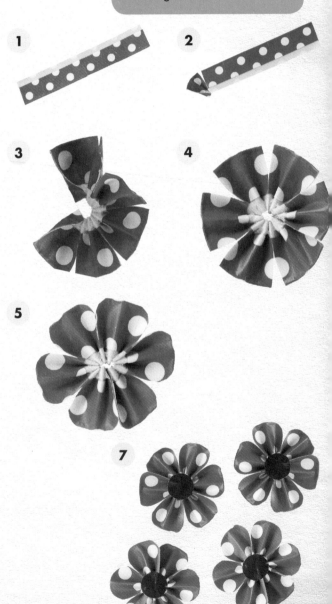

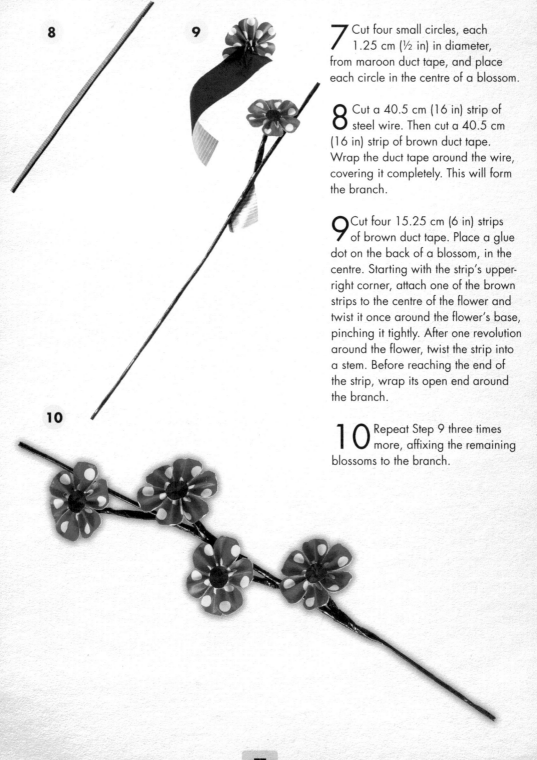

8

9

10

7 Cut four small circles, each 1.25 cm (½ in) in diameter, from maroon duct tape, and place each circle in the centre of a blossom.

8 Cut a 40.5 cm (16 in) strip of steel wire. Then cut a 40.5 cm (16 in) strip of brown duct tape. Wrap the duct tape around the wire, covering it completely. This will form the branch.

9 Cut four 15.25 cm (6 in) strips of brown duct tape. Place a glue dot on the back of a blossom, in the centre. Starting with the strip's upper-right corner, attach one of the brown strips to the centre of the flower and twist it once around the flower's base, pinching it tightly. After one revolution around the flower, twist the strip into a stem. Before reaching the end of the strip, wrap its open end around the branch.

10 Repeat Step 9 three times more, affixing the remaining blossoms to the branch.

60. White Peony

Materials

» White duct tape
» Green duct tape
» Yellow duct tape

Additional Tools

» Thin black marker

1 Cut a 56-cm (22-in) long strip of white duct tape. With its sticky side facing upward, fold the strip inward lengthwise so that only a 6.5 mm (¼ in) strip of the sticky side remains exposed. Add one more strip to the bottom.

2 Pull up one end and wind the strip around itself with its sticky side facing inward. Pinch the sticky end, and allow some space between the layers.

3 When the full length of the strip has been wound into the shape of a flower's head, pinch the sticky end tightly to ensure that it won't come apart.

4 Cut a 25.5-cm (10-in) long strip of green duct tape, and cut a 7.5 cm (3 in) row of 'V'-shaped pieces, working inward along its top edge from its top right corner.

5 Carefully pry up the strip and, starting with its upper right edge, wrap the green strip around the bottom of the flower; the peaks of the 'V'-shapes should point upward toward the flower's petals. After circling the flower head once, twist the green strip downward into a stem.

6 Use the detail scissors to cut small, gently-curved ridges into the top edges of the petals. Make regular downward cuts from the dip of every second ridge down to the base of the flower.

7 Cut smaller, wedge-shaped gaps into the edges of these petals 1.5 mm (¹⁄₁₆ in) wide at the top. Fluff out the petals.

8 Cut a 6.5 mm (¼ in) square from the yellow duct tape, and place it in the flower's centre.

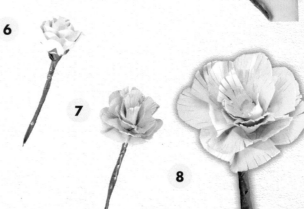

1
2
3
4
5
6
7
8

Materials

» Hot pink duct tape
» White duct tape
» Lime green duct tape
» Two small pieces of scrap paper

Additional Tools

» Pencil

1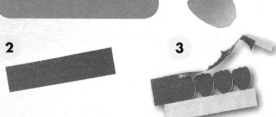

2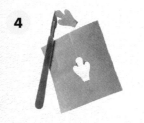

3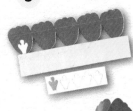

4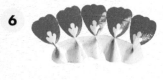

5

6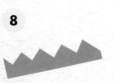

7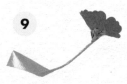

8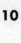

9

10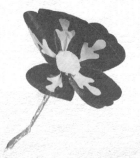

61. Hot Pink Hibiscus

1 Create a symmetrical petal template by first folding a piece of scrap paper in half. Draw half of a petal, with the fold as a vertical dividing line, 7.5 cm (3 in) tall and (folded) 3.25 cm (1¼ in) wide.

2 Make a double-sided layered fabric with hot pink duct tape 30.5 cm (12 in) wide and 7.5 cm (3 in) high; ensure that the folded edge is positioned at the top, and leave the bottom edge unfinished with a sticky edge facing downward. Add another strip of hot pink duct tape along the bottom edge.

3 Lay the fabric sticky-side-up and place the unfolded petal template on top, just above the sticky strip. Trace five petals, with each touching the side edge of the next. Cut out these petals, but leave them attached to the duct tape fabric at the bottom.

4 Create a template for the white shape of the inner flower petal by again folding a piece of scrap paper vertically in half and drawing one side of a shape like a small ghost with two raised hands, 5 cm (2 in) tall and, folded, 1.25 cm (½ in) wide.

5 Cut a 18-cm (7-in) long strip of white duct tape, and trace five inner petal shapes onto it. Cut them out with a craft knife and affix each to the lower centre of each hibiscus petal.

(Continued overleaf)

6 Pinch the base of each hibiscus petal from the back, folding the sticky lip of duct tape below in on itself.

7 Twist the sticky strip at the bottom tightly, bringing the petals together in the centre.

8 Place an 20.5 cm (8 in) strip of lime green duct tape on the cutting mat, sticky side down. Cut 'V'-shaped pieces out of its top edge.

9 Pull this strip up and, with its pointed edge facing upward, use it to cover the twisted outside portion of the hibiscus flower's base. Twist and wrap the lime green duct tape onto itself at a 45-degree downward angle, so that it tapers into a stem.

10 Cut out a white duct tape circle with a 2.5 cm (1 in) diameter, and affix the circle to the centre of the flower.

62. Orchid

1 Cut an 20.5-cm (8-in) long strip of white duct tape, and, with its sticky side facing upward, fold over a 6.5 mm (¼ in) lip lengthwise from its bottom edge. Place a second strip of white duct tape on top of it, overlapping its top edge by 6.5 mm (¼ in).

2 Create a stencil for the inner petal. Shaped like the spade symbol in a deck of cards, it should be equal in height to the combined white strips, with a narrow 'handle' 6.5 mm (¼ in) high. Trace this stencil twice onto the white fabric; draw its handles onto the sticky overlapping strip. Cut out both shapes.

3 Cut the remaining portion of the white strip into three 2.5 cm (1 in) wide rectangles.

4 Fold one rectangle inward so that its left and right sides meet, and with its sticky side facing outward. Fold the outer edges back toward the middle, creating an accordion fold. Pinch its sticky base to make this fold permanent. Do the same to the other two rectangles.

5 Connect the two large inner petals at their base, and attach the three rectangles around the petals at their bases at evenly-spaced intervals, so that their outer edges fan out. Pinch the base tightly to secure the petals together.

1

2

3

4
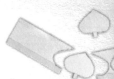

5
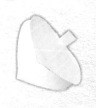

Materials

» White duct tape
» Green duct tape
» Hot pink duct tape
» Scrap paper for template

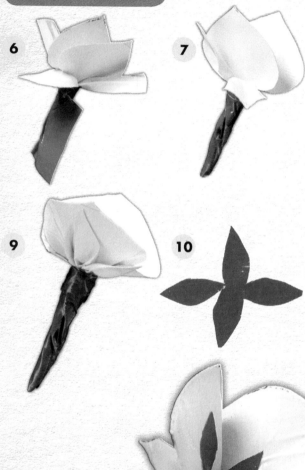

6 Cut a 10-cm (4-in) long strip of green duct tape and affix one of its ends to the outer base of the flower. Pinching it tightly, roll the strip around the base of the flower twice before twisting it downward into a short stem.

7 Use scissors to shape the tips of the three outer petals so that they curve and taper into points.

8 Cut a 10-cm (4-in) long strip of green duct tape and cut it down to a 1.25 cm (½ in) width.

9 Push the inner petals outward from the centre to round out the flower, and simultaneously press the base upward. Tightly wrap the green strip round the flower's base to secure this shape.

10 Cut a 3.75-cm (1½-in) long strip of hot pink duct tape, and trim it into a small, four-petal flower shape measuring 2.5 cm (1 in) square. Affix this shape to the centre of the inner petals.

63. Iris

Materials

» Blue duct tape
» White duct tape
» Yellow duct tape
» Green duct tape

1 Cut an 20.5-cm (8-in) long strip of blue duct tape. With its sticky side facing upward, fold its bottom edge upward to make a 6.5 mm (¼ in) high blue lip. Place a second strip of blue duct tape on top of it, overlapping its top edge by 6.5 mm (¼ in).

2 With the sticky side facing inward, wind the strip around itself for roughly two and a half revolutions. Pinch the sticky end together as you go, and allow some space between the layers. Give the strip's sticky end a few tight pinches to ensure it won't come apart. This forms the basic shape of the flower's head.

3 Cut a 30.5-cm (12-in) long strip of green duct tape, and affix one end to the outer base of the flower. Pinch the base tightly, and roll the strip round the base of the flower twice before twisting it downward into a long stem.

4 Cut the flower's outer edge into three petal shapes, then three more petals on the inner circle 6.5 mm (¼ in) shorter.

5 Cut two 10 cm (4 in) strips of duct tape, one yellow and one white. Cut out three white triangles 1.25 cm (½ in) wide and 3.75 cm (1½ in) high. Then cut three yellow triangles 1.25 cm (½ in) wide and 2.5 cm (1 in) high, and affix them to the white triangles, aligning their bottom edges.

6 Pull each of the flower's outer petals downward and affix one of the combined white and yellow triangles to each petal, points facing outward. Then push the outer petals back up.

7 Repeat Step 3 to reinforce the flower's stem.

8 Pull down the outer circle of petals again.

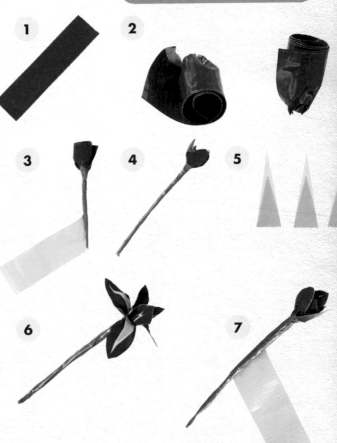

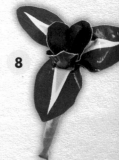

Materials

» Yellow duct tape
» Lime green duct tape

Additional Tools

» Detail scissors

64. Yellow Tulip

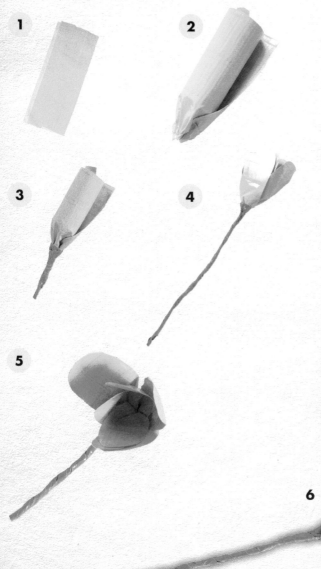

1 Use yellow duct tape to make a double-sided layer fabric 30.5 cm (12 in) wide by 12.5 cm (5 in) high; leave an exposed sticky strip at least 1.25 cm (½ in) high.

2 With the sticky side facing inward, roll the fabric lengthwise for two revolutions. Pinch the strip's sticky end as you twist it, and allow some space between each of the layers.

4 Cut a 25.5-cm (10-in) long strip of lime green duct tape. Wrap the length of the strip tightly round the flower's base, then after one revolution twist the green strip tightly to form the stem.

5 Use detail scissors to cut out eight tongue-shaped petals, four from each of the yellow strip's two revolutions.

6 Once all eight petals are cut out, push the petals inward toward the centre.

CHAPTER 7:

Toys for Kids

There's something about the novelty of duct tape that appeals to children of all ages. A brand new roll of the stuff can conjure up imagined scents and flavors, like walking into a candy shop. The hot pink spools can be watermelon lollipops with chewy centres, and the bright yellow reels can be banana-flavored jellybeans. Kids are driven by their curiosity, wanting to experience the world through their senses of sight and touch and taste first.

There's an immediate euphoric reaction when you tell them, 'Hey, that's made out of duct tape'. It's as if you upended their expectations and surprised them. Toys made from duct tape are great gifts, and these projects are a sure bet to make any kid smile.

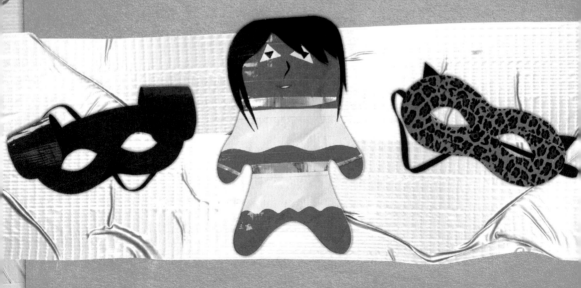

Materials
» Black duct tape
» White duct tape
» Silver duct tape

65. Chess/ Draughts Board

1

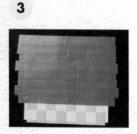

2

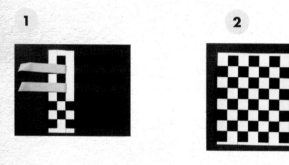

3

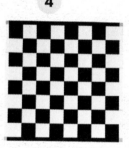

4

5

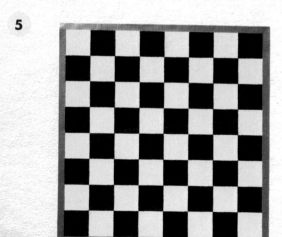

1 Make a 40.5 cm (16 in) square woven fabric. To create the green-and-white chequer pattern, cut eight 43 cm (17 in) strips of black duct tape first and arrange them consecutively on the cutting mat in the horizontal position. Then cut eight 43 cm (17 in) strips of white duct tape and weave them into the black tape, one strip at a time. When beginning the weave, be sure to leave an approximately 1.25 cm (½ in) border on the outer edge.

2 Square up the sides, but be sure to allow for 1.25 cm (½ in) border outside of the chequer pattern. Gently pry one corner with the craft knife and slowly pull up by hand in a firm diagonal motion.

3 Place fabric on the cutting mat with the sticky side facing up. Cover with strips of silver duct tape. Be sure the strips overlap each other by at least 1.5 mm (1/16 in).

4 Flip over and trim the excess silver duct tape on all four sides.

5 Cut two 40.5 cm (16 in) strips of silver duct tape. The cut each strip lengthwise in half. Take each strip and cover the 1.25 cm (½ in) border on every side of the chequer design. Flip over. Finish the edges by folding the silver duct tape strips down. Cut off any excess duct tape at the corners.

66. Blue Boy Doll

Materials

» Brown paper
» Royal blue duct tape
» White duct tape
» Black duct tape
» Red duct tape
» Metallic silver duct tape
» Fibrefill

Additional Tools

» White grease pencil

1 Create a doll template (this can also be used for the Pink Girl Doll in the following project). Vertically fold the brown paper bag in half. Draw one side of a very simplistic body (half a head, half a torso, one arm, one leg) approximately 30.5 cm (12 in) high. Make sure the edges are rounded and there are no sharp corners. Cut out shape and unfold.

2 Using the royal blue duct tape, make a single-sided layer fabric large enough for your doll template to fit inside of.

3 Trace the outline of the doll onto the fabric and cut out the shape.

4 Pry the top edge with the craft knife and pull up by hand. Flip over so the sticky side is facing up. Place small pieces of fibrefill on top and try to stay within the lines of the doll shape. Put just enough fibrefill to cover the sticky surface, rather than piling it on.

5 Starting from the top cover the doll shape with strips of royal blue duct tape. Be sure to overlap by at least $\frac{1}{16}$ in. (1.5 mm). As you cover the doll shape with the strips, stop every two strips and add a little more fibrefill to the inside.

6 Once you've covered the entire doll shape, flip over. Trim the

1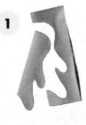

3

4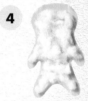

5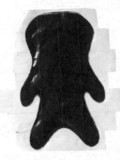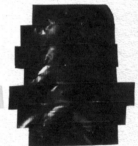

6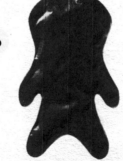

7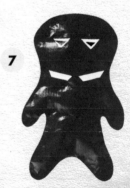

excess duct tape. Press down in the nooks and small spaces along the outline of the doll, especially underneath the arms. If there are openings or gaps, close them up with small strips of royal blue duct tape.

7 Make a face for the doll. Cut out two triangles from a strip of white duct tape. Place them on the upper portion of the doll head, upside down so the wide bases are the top edges and the apexes are at the bottom. These are the eyes – cut two smaller triangles from black duct tape and affix these inside them as pupils. Then cut out two small trapezoids from the white duct tape and place them upside down around the neck of the doll. This is the shirt collar.

8 From the red duct tape cut out a small tongue and place it in the centre of the head, close to the neck. Take a small piece of white duct tape and cut out a small triangle. Place the triangle on the upper right top edge of the tongue. This is the snaggle-tooth.

9 Cut out a slight crescent for the nose and a small wave shape for

the mouth. Place them on the doll face.

10 To make the necktie, cut out a skinny and tall pentagon approximately 1.25 cm (½ in) wide and 5 cm (2 in) high from the silver chrome duct tape. The triangular top should be slightly wider than the base. Turn it around so the triangular top is at the bottom. Place it on the doll, the flat base positioned in between the two collar pieces. Then cut a 1.25 cm (½ in) square from the silver chrome duct tape and place it on top of the pentagon base, which is positioned in between the two collar pieces. This is the knot of the necktie.

10

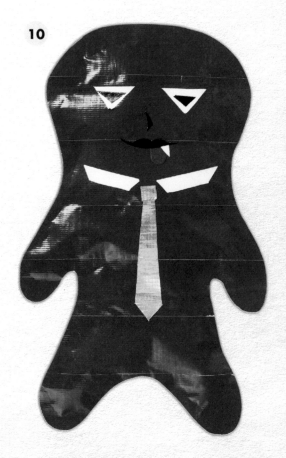

8

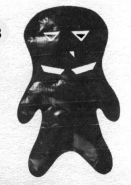

67. Pink Girl Doll

Materials

» Brown paper
» Hot pink duct tape
» White duct tape
» Red duct tape
» Black duct tape
» Metallic silver duct tape
» Fibrefill

Additional Tools

» White grease pencil

1 Create a doll template (See Step 1 from the previous project). Vertically fold the brown paper bag in half. Draw one side of a very simplistic body (half a head, half a torso, one arm, one leg) approximately 30.5 cm (12 in) high. Make sure the edges are rounded and there are no sharp corners. Cut out the shape and unfold.

2 Using the hot pink duct tape make a single-sided layer fabric large enough for your doll template to fit inside of. Trace the outline of the doll onto the fabric and cut out the shape.

3 Pry the top edge with the craft knife and pull up by hand. Flip over so the sticky side is facing up. Place small pieces of fibrefill on top and try to stay within the lines of the doll shape. Put just enough fibrefill to cover the sticky surface. Do not pile it on.

4 Starting from the top cover the doll shape with strips of hot pink duct tape. Be sure to overlap by at least 1.5 mm ($\frac{1}{16}$ in). As you cover the doll shape with the strips, stop every two strips and add a little more fibrefill to the inside.

5 Once you've covered the entire doll shape, flip over. Trim the excess duct tape. Press down in the nooks and small spaces along the outline of the doll, especially underneath the arms. If there are openings or gaps, close them up with small strips of hot pink duct tape.

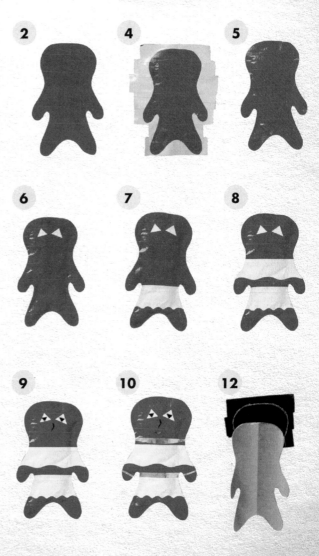

6 Make a face. Cut out two triangles from a strip of white duct tape. Place them on the upper portion of the doll head with wide bases on the bottom and the apexes at the top. These are the eyes.

7 Create a skirt. Overlap two 12.5 cm (5 in) strips of duct tape. Place the doll template on top and trace the sides with white grease pencil, from the hips down to the knees. Remove the template and cut along the lines to make a skirt. Make scalloped edges at the bottom. Gently pry the top edge with the craft knife and pull up by hand. Place the skirt on the doll.

8 Create a blouse. Overlap two 12.5 cm (5 in) strips of duct tape. Place the doll template on top and trace the sides with white grease pencil, from the neck down to the wrists. Remove the template and cut along the lines to make a blouse. Make scalloped edges at the bottom. Gently pry the top edge with the craft knife and pull up by hand. Place skirt on the doll.

9 Cut two small triangles from black duct tape. Place them inside the eyes of the doll. These are the pupils of the eyes. Cut out a slight crescent for the nose and place it on the doll's face.

10 Cut tiny bands out of a strip of silver chrome duct tape. Place them round the wrists for bracelets. Cut a wider band, approximately 1.25 cm (½ in) wide. Place it on the waist for the belt. Cut a narrow ellipse and place it on the neck for a necklace. Trim off any excess duct tape. Cut out a pair of lips from the red duct tape. Place it on the face below the nose. Then cut a sliver of white and place it on top of the lips for teeth.

11 Using the black duct tape make a double-sided layer fabric measuring 17.75 cm (7 in) wide by 11.5 cm (4½ in) tall. Place a strip of black duct tape across the top edge, leaving approximately half of the strip lengthwise with an exposed sticky side facing down.

12 Take the doll template and trace the head onto the black duct tape with the white grease pencil.

13 Using the head outline as a rough guide, cut out the shape of hair for the doll. Gently pry an edge with the craft knife and pull up by hand. Place hair on the doll.

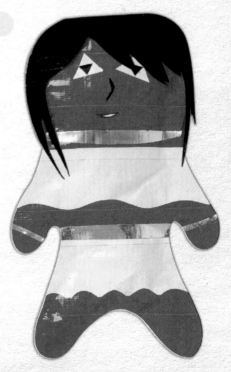

Masks

For all masks (projects 68–72), begin by tracing a mask template onto scrap paper, then cut it out with a craft knife.

To finish, place a glue dot at each end of an elastic band, then attach its ends to the back left and right sides of the mask. Cover each end with small strips of matching-coloured duct tape.

Materials

» At least two colours of duct tape
» 20.5 cm x 10 cm (8 in x 4 in) scrap paper
» 20.5 cm (8 in) strip of elastic band, 6.5 mm (¼ in) wide
» Glue dots

Additional Tools

» White grease pencil
» Black permanent marker

68. Elephant Mask

1 Using silver duct tape and hot pink duct tape, make a double-sided layer fabric measuring at least 21.5 cm (8½ in) wide by 11.5 cm (4½ in) high. Make one side entirely silver and the other hot pink.

2 Trace the mask template onto the fabric with a white grease pencil, then cut out the shape from the fabric.

3 Make another double-sided layer fabric 31.75 cm (12½ in) wide by 20.5 cm (8 in) high, with one side silver and the other hot pink. Trace the ear and trunk templates onto the silver side of the fabric with a white grease pencil, and cut out the shapes with a craft knife.

4 Attach the ears to the sides of the mask with glue dots. Attach the trunk to the middle of the mask right below the eye, and draw wrinkles across it with a black permanent marker.

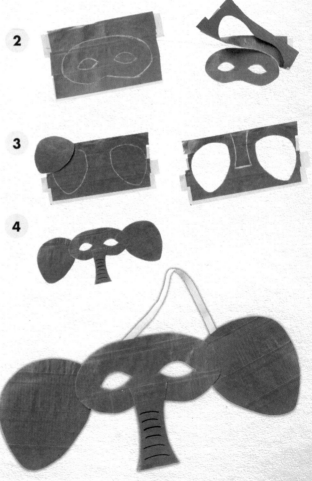

69. **Leopard Mask**

1 Make a double-sided layered duct tape fabric 21.5 cm (8½ in) wide by 11.5 cm (4½ in) high, with one side leopard print and the other black.

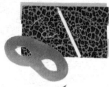

2 Trace the mask template onto the fabric with a white grease pencil and cut out the shape. Save the elliptical pieces from inside the eye-holes, but discard the rest.

3 Place the mask template on top of the cut-out fabric upside down so that the notch for the nose is on top of the mask's forehead. Trace this notch onto the mask and cut along this line with a craft knife.

4 Cut off the bottom third of each of the two elliptical pieces and affix one to each side of the mask's top edge on the reverse, using small strips of black duct tape. These are the ears.

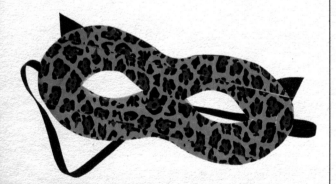

70. **Zebra Mask**

1 Make a double-sided layered duct tape fabric 21.5 cm (8½ in) wide by 11.5 cm (4½ in) high, with one side zebra print and the other black.

2 Trace the mask template onto the fabric with a white grease pencil and cut out the shape. Save the elliptical pieces from inside the eye-holes, but discard the rest.

3 Attach these elliptical pieces to the top of the mask with glue dots, one on each side, with their black sides facing outward. These are the ears.

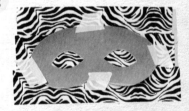

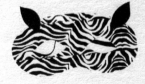

71. Cat Mask

1 Using white duct tape and hot pink duct tape, make a double-sided layer fabric measuring at least 21.5 cm (8½ in) wide by 11.5 cm (4½ in) high. Make one side entirely white and the other hot pink. Trace the mask template onto the fabric with a white grease pencil.

2 Cut out the mask from the fabric. Save the elliptical pieces from the inside of the eyes. Discard the rest.

3 Cut out a curved triangle from a piece of hot pink duct tape. Rotate the mask so the nose notch is at the top and the forehead is at the bottom. This is the right way up for the cat mask. Place the hot pink triangle on the bottom centre.

4 Cut off the bottom third of each ear. Attach them to the top of the mask with small strips of hot pink duct tape, one on each side, with their white sides facing upward. These are the ears.

5 Cut a 30.5 cm (12 in) strip of black duct tape. Fold it onto itself, aligning the outer edges as much as possible, and leaving a 1.25 cm (½ in) strip of the sticky surface open at one end.

6 Cut the black duct tape into six 3.25 mm (⅛ in) strips. These are the whiskers: attach three to each side of the nose.

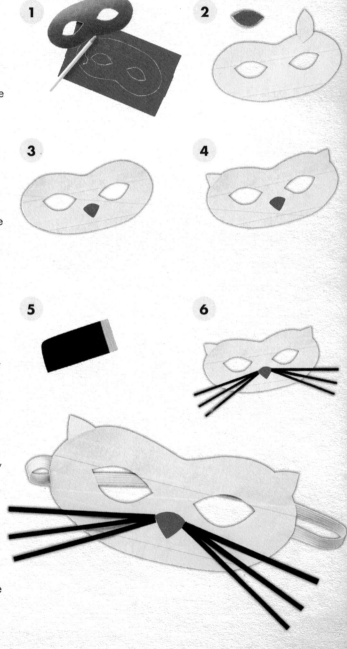

72. Dog Mask

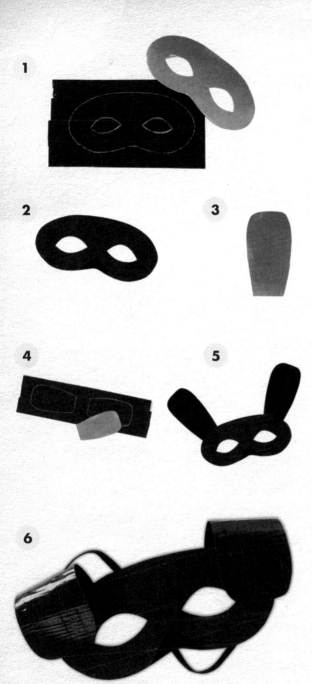

1 Make a double-sided layered duct tape fabric 21.5 cm (8½ in) wide by 11.5 cm (4½ in) high, with one side brown and the other black. Trace the mask template onto the fabric with a white grease pencil and cut out the shape.

2 Cut a triangle from black duct tape, 5 cm (2 in) wide at its base, 2.5 cm (1 in) high, and with a 90-degree angle at its apex. Affix this black triangle just above the mask's nose notch, and trim it to follow the mask's outline.

3 Make a template for the dog's ears, 11.5 cm (4½ in) high by 6.5 cm (2½ in) wide. The ears should be rounded at the top and taper inward toward the base.

4 Make a double-sided layer fabric 30.5 cm (12 in) wide by 9 cm (3½ in) high, one side brown and the other black. Trace the ear template onto the fabric twice with a white grease pencil.

5 Cut out the ear shapes from the fabric and, with their black sides facing outward, attach one to each top side of the mask with small pieces of black duct tape.

6 Place a glue dot on the top of each ear, bend them downward and affix them to the sides of the eyes.

73. Skipping Rope

Materials

» Lime green duct tape
» Orange duct tape

1 Cut a 91.5-cm (36-in) long strip of orange duct tape, and lay it on the cutting mat sticky-side-up. Fold its bottom edge up and over to make a 6.5 mm (¼ in) orange border.

2 Keep folding the bottom edge up and over the first fold, until a cord is formed.

3 Repeat Steps 1 through 3 twice more, so that you have three orange cords. Cut a strip of orange duct tape measuring 6.5 cm (2½ in) long. Cut it in half lengthwise.

4 Pull up one of the small tape strips and place it on the cutting mat sticky-side-up. Place the ends of two orange cords on top, end to end, and fold the strip over to join them. Do the same with the remaining tape strip to attach one end of the two connected cords to the third one. All three cords should now be connected, forming a single cord 274 cm (108 in) long.

5 Repeat Steps 1 to 4 using lime green duct tape, so that you have two 274 cm (108 in) long cords: one orange, one lime green.

6 Hold the cords together and tie a single knot at one end. Make a second knot 12.5 cm (5 in) further down, to form one of the handles.

7 Hold the handle down on the cutting mat with a small piece of duct tape, and twist the loose cords together.

8 Tie a third knot approximately 12.5 cm (5 in) from the end of the open cords, then make a fourth knot as close to the end of the cords as possible to form the second handle.

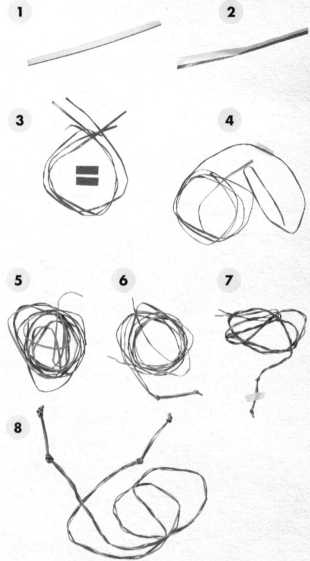

Materials

» Putty duct tape
» Black duct tape
» Silver chrome duct tape
» Gold chrome duct tape
» White duct tape

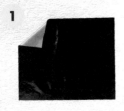

74. Backgammon Board

1 Make a double-sided layered fabric 52 cm (20 in) wide by 40.5 cm (16 in) high, using black duct tape for the front side and putty tape for the reverse side. Square up the sides.

2 Cut a strip of white duct tape 40.5 cm (16 in) long, then cut a 1.25 cm (½ in) wide strip from it. Affix this strip to the board vertically up its middle. This is known as the bar of the board.

3 Mark 16.5 cm (6½ in) upward from the bottom corners on the board's left and right edges with a white grease pencil. Draw a horizontal line between both marks.

4 Cut two 23-cm (9-in) long strips of duct tape, one silver and one gold. Cut a straight line diagonally across the strip from its bottom left corner to its top right corner, to create four triangles.

5 Affix one silver triangle to the left edge of the board, with its pointed apex touching the 16.5 cm (6½ in) high horizontal line and the left edge of its base approximately 6.5 mm (¼ in) from the board's left edge. Affix one gold triangle to the board with its base approximately 3.25 mm (⅛ in) from the right side of the silver triangle, and with its apex touching the horizontal line.

(continued overleaf)

1

2
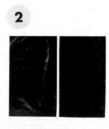

3
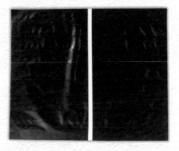

4

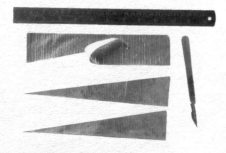

5
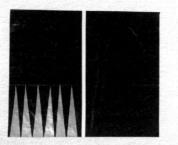

6 Pry the edge of the remaining silver triangle with the craft knife and pull up by hand. Place the triangle down with the skinny apex touching the 16.5 cm (6½ in) high horizontal line and the base approximately 3.25 mm (⅛ in) from the right side of the gold triangle.

7 Pull up the remaining silver triangle and place it on the board with its base approximately 3.25 mm (⅛ in) from the right side of the gold triangle, with its apex vertically aligned with those of the other two triangles. Do the same with the remaining gold triangle, placing it 3.25 mm (⅛ in) from the right edge of the last silver triangle.

8 Repeat Step 4 twice, then continue to add triangles along the bottom edge, alternating silver and gold. There should be six triangles on each side of the white bar, so twelve in total. Trim the excess tape along the bottom edge with the metal ruler and craft knife.

9 Rotate board 180 degrees, and repeat Steps 4 through 8 on the other side of the board. There should now be twenty-four triangles on the completed board.

9

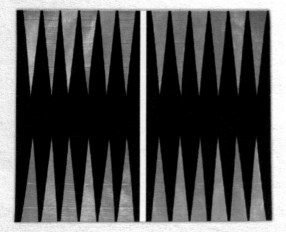

75. Boat

1 Make a striped double-sided layered fabric 46 cm (18 in) wide by 30.5 cm (12 in) high. Square up the sides.

2 With the stripes vertically orientated, pull the top edge down toward the bottom edge and fold the fabric in half. Run the bone folder along the crease for a tighter fold.

3 Fold one of the top left and right corners downward toward the vertical centre, forming a triangular apex at the top. Run the bone folder along these folds.

4 Fold the bottom edges upward, making a horizontal fold where it meets the folded edges created in Step 3. This forms a cuff. Fold the top left and right corners of the cuff over, to follow the 90-degree angles of the top edges.

5 Flip the boat over from right to left and repeat Step 4. You should have a straightforward triangle.

6 The bottom edge of the triangle should now open into a pocket. Hold the bottom left and right corners and slide a finger inside, then pull the corners toward each other so the pocket opens and the corners meet up. The shape should change into a square.

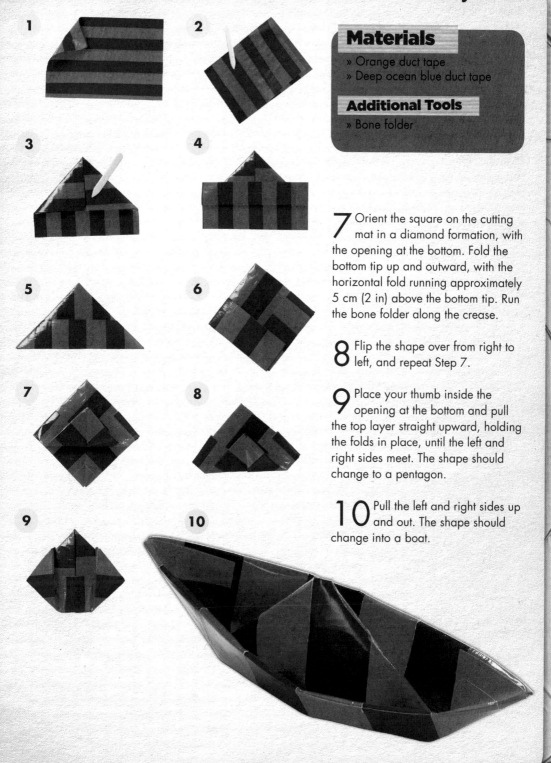

1

2

Materials
» Orange duct tape
» Deep ocean blue duct tape

Additional Tools
» Bone folder

3

4

7 Orient the square on the cutting mat in a diamond formation, with the opening at the bottom. Fold the bottom tip up and outward, with the horizontal fold running approximately 5 cm (2 in) above the bottom tip. Run the bone folder along the crease.

5

6

8 Flip the shape over from right to left, and repeat Step 7.

7

8

9 Place your thumb inside the opening at the bottom and pull the top layer straight upward, holding the folds in place, until the left and right sides meet. The shape should change to a pentagon.

9

10

10 Pull the left and right sides up and out. The shape should change into a boat.

CHAPTER 8:

Costumes, Disguises and Props

The idea of homemade costumes is nothing new. Often constructed with some cardboard, a little tape and a lot of imagination, they trump any store-bought outfit. As a child I loved making my own Hallowe'en costumes, and as a parent I love making them for my own kids. My son was obsessed with locomotives, so I made him rocket, tugboat and train costumes. The most memorable costume I made for my daughter was a tree, complete with leaves and branches.

Sometimes it takes a few tries to get it right, but the beauty of these duct tape costumes, disguises and props is their resilience. Duct tape is a material that can withstand inclement weather as well as the mishandling of children and uncoordinated adults alike. A spilled drink is not the end of the world. That ketchup drip does not mean the costume is ruined. And let it rain, baby! A damp sponge or a towel is all you need to make things right again.

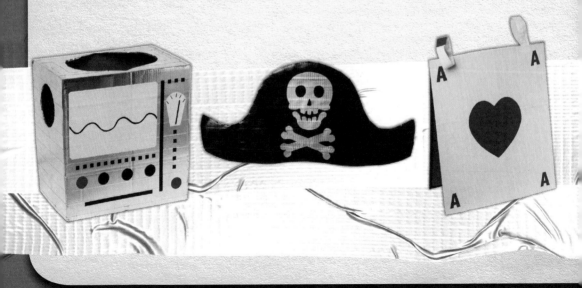

Materials

» Black duct tape
» Piece of scrap paper at least 26.5 cm (10½ in) wide by 15.25 cm (6 in) high
» 25.5 cm (10 in) of elastic band, 1.25 cm (½ in) wide
» Glue dots

76. Glossy Beard

1 Draw a beard stencil, sized appropriately, on the scrap paper and cut it out.

2 Use black duct tape to make a double-sided layered fabric at least 26.5 cm (10½ in) wide by 15.25 cm (6 in) high. Trace the beard stencil onto the fabric using a white grease pencil and cut out the shape.

3 Place a glue dot on the right tip of the beard, and place one end of the elastic band on top of the glue dot. Cover it with a piece of duct tape and trim any excess.

4 Repeat Step 3 for the left tip of the beard so that the band is secured on both sides, and the beard is ready to wear.

2
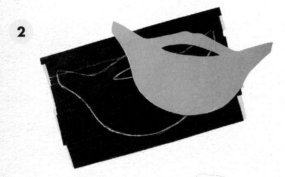

3

4
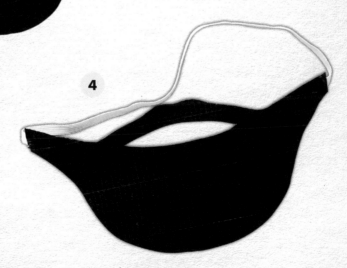

77. Superhero Cape

Materials
» Deep ocean blue duct tape
» Red duct tape
» Silver chrome duct tape

Additional Tools
» White grease pencil
» Hole puncher, with a diameter of 3.25 to 6.5 mm (⅛ to ¼ in)

1 Make three double-sided layered fabrics 86.5 cm (34 in) wide by 30.5 cm (12 in) high, using deep ocean blue duct tape for the front sides and red for the reverse sides. Combine the three pieces along their 86.5 cm (34 in) wide sides with strips of matching duct tape, creating a single fabric measuring 86.5 x 91.5 cm (34 in.x 36 in).

2 Fold the combined fabric in half so it measures 86.5 cm x 45.5 cm (34 in x 18 in), and position it with the folded edge on the left side. On the top edge measure and mark 18.5 cm (7¼ in) inward from the top left corner with the white grease pencil. Draw a straight diagonal line between these two marks, then cut along the line with scissors. Gently round the bottom corner.

3 Draw a horizontal line across the cape 3.75 cm (1½ in) downward from its top edge, then mark off every centimeter (2/5 in). Use the hole puncher to cut holes through both layers at each of these marks.

4 Cut a 61 cm (24 in) strip of silver chrome duct tape, then halve the strip lengthwise. Twist both halves into thin ropes, then join the two pieces to form one long rope.

5 Cut into one end of the rope at an angle to make it pointed. Weave the rope through the holes along the top edge of the cape. Cinch this edge to make the cape rounded – this part is worn around the neck.

6 Make a one-sided layered fabric with silver chrome duct tape, on top of baking paper. Cut out a large single letter or symbol, and some star stickers. Use these stickers to decorate

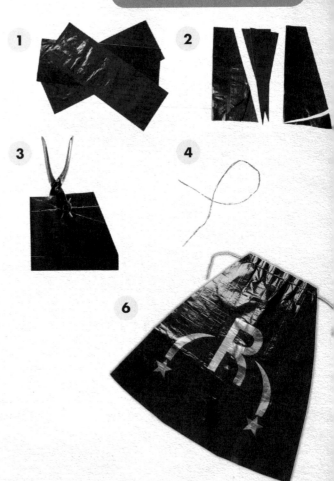

78. Pirate Hat

Materials

» Black duct tape
» Silver duct tape
» Gold chrome duct tape
» Piece of scrap paper, at least 48.5 cm x 25.5 cm (19 in x 10 in)

Additional Tools

» White grease pencil

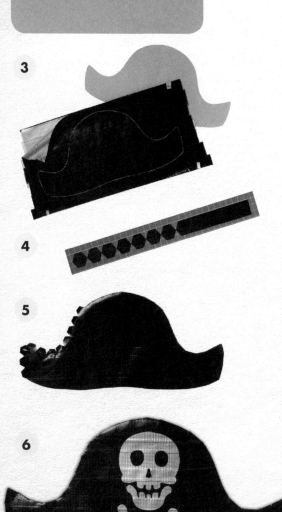

3

4

5

6

1 Draw and cut out a hat template with scrap paper. To ensure a good fit, make the hat's width, discounting the brim, slightly more than half the circumference of the wearer's head.

2 Make two double-sided layered fabrics with front sides black and reverses silver, with both at least a centimeter (2/5 in) taller and wider than the hat stencil.

3 Place one fabric on the cutting mat silver side up, then place the other on top with its black side facing upward; secure them in place with small tape strips. Trace the hat template onto the top fabric with the white grease pencil, then cut the shape out of both fabrics.

4 Cut a 30.5 cm (12 in) strip of black duct tape, then halve it lengthwise. On each strip make 'X'-shaped cuts every 2.5 cm (1 in), to create hexagon-shaped pieces.

5 Use these hexagons of tape to seal the top and side seams between the two hat-shaped fabrics, with the outer points of the hexagon meeting along the seam. Leave the bottom edge open; this completes the main hat.

6 To create the Jolly Roger sticker, see the instructions on page 51.

79. Knight's Sword

Materials

» Silver chrome duct tape
» Black duct tape
» Piece of corrugated board at least 25.5 cm (10 in) wide by 61 cm (24 in) high
» Glue dots

Additional Tools

» Black marker pen

1 Cut a piece of corrugated board measuring 5 cm (2 in) wide and 61 cm (24 in) long. Cut with, rather than across, the grain of the corrugated board, parallel with the ridges, as this will make the blade of the sword stronger. Cut one end into a point.

2 Cut a support piece out of corrugated board measuring 2.5 cm (1 in) wide and 30.5 cm (12 in) long; again, cut with the grain. Attach this piece to the blade with glue dots, placing one end of it 3.75 cm (1½ in) from the bottom (flat) edge. Cover the reinforced blade with silver chrome duct tape.

3 Cut a piece of corrugated board 25.5 cm (10 in) wide by 15.5 cm (6 in) high, and draw a vertical line down its middle with a black marker. Draw a horizontal line across the board 3.75 cm (1½ in) down from its top edge. Measure 3.75 cm (1½ in) inward from the left edge and draw a vertical line downward from the horizontal one, then another vertical line 3.75 cm (1½ in) to the right of the middle vertical line. There should now be a 'T'-shape on the corrugated board's left side.

4 Cut this board in half along the middle vertical line. Place the left half on top of the other half, then cut out the 'T'-shape from both pieces of board.

1

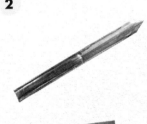

2

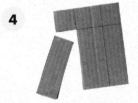

3

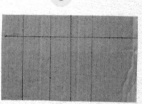

4

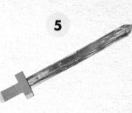

5

5 Attach one panel of the 'T'-shaped handle to the base of the blade with glue dots, so it sits directly below the blade support.

6 Use the excess pieces of board from Step 4 as spacers between the handle panels. With the back panel beneath the blade, affix the spacers to the inside of the handle using glue dots.

7 Attach the front panel of the handle to the spacers with glue dots. Be sure to line up the edges to the back panel of the handle. Cover the handle with black duct tape.

6

7

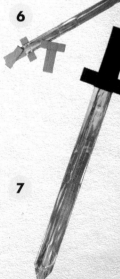

Materials

» Silver chrome duct tape
» Black duct tape
» Red duct tape
» Brown paper
» A piece of corrugated board at least 40.5 cm (16 in) wide by 61 cm (24 in) high

80. Knight's Shield

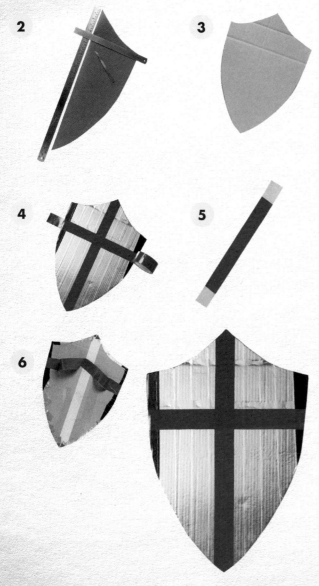

1 Trim a piece of brown paper to measure 24 in. (61 cm) high and 16 in. (40.5 cm) wide. Fold it in half from right to left, so that its width is 8 in (20.5 cm).

2 Measure and mark 4 in. (10 cm) downward from the top right corner. Use the craft knife to cut a slightly rounded, concave diagonal line from the top left corner to the 4 in. (10 cm) mark on the right edge. Then, from that same mark, cut a slightly rounded, convex diagonal line. Unfold the brown paper – this is the complete shield template.

3 Trace the outline of the shield onto the corrugated board, then cut out the shape.

4 Cover the shield with silver chrome duct tape, then place a vertical strip of black duct tape down its left and right sides. Place two strips of red duct tape – one horizontal, one vertical – across the centre of the shield.

5 Cut a 51 cm (20 in) strip of red duct tape, and lay it down sticky-side-up. Cut a 38-cm (15-in) long strip of red duct tape, and place this shorter strip on top of the longer one, centred. This will form the strap.

6 Attach the strap to the reverse side of the shield with its exposed sticky ends.

81. Robot

1 Assemble the top of the box, taping the sides together with silver duct tape. Use the craft knife to cut a hole in the top side (the side with flaps) large enough to fit your head through, at least 30.5 cm (12 in) in diameter.

2 On one side of the box measure 5 cm (2 in) down from the top edge, then use a compass to draw a circle with a diameter measuring 14 cm (5½ in) in the centre of that same side; the top of the circle should touch the 5 cm (2 in) mark. Use the craft knife to cut out the circle. This is an armhole.

3 Repeat Step 2 to create a second armhole on the opposite side of the box. Cover the entire box with silver chrome duct tape, but leave the bottom end open.

4 Affix one strip of black duct tape and one of red duct tape to a piece of baking paper. Use a plastic bottle cap to trace circles onto both of the strips with a white grease pencil. Cut these circles out and set them aside; they will be used as button stickers.

5 Cut another strip of black duct tape, then cut it into thinner 1.25-cm (½-in) wide strips. Set these aside.

Materials

» Silver chrome duct tape
» White duct tape
» Black duct tape
» Red duct tape
» A corrugated cardboard box, flat, approximately 45.5 cm x 45.5 cm x 45.5 cm (18 in x 18 in x 18 in)

Additional Tools

» Compass
» Plastic bottle caps
» Brown paper
» Baking paper

1

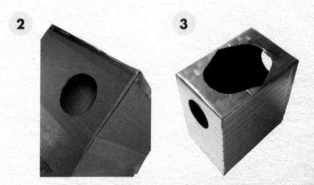

2

3

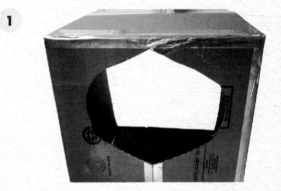

5

6

10

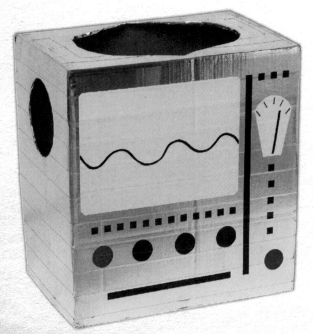

6 Make a one-sided layered white duct tape fabric on top of parchment paper, measuring at least 28 cm (11 in) wide by 30.5 cm (12 in) high. Cut out a rectangle 25.5 cm (10 in) wide by 20.5 cm (8 in) high, and round the corners. This will be a computer screen. Then, cut a lightbulb-shaped piece with straight sides – this will be a meter reader.

7 Remove the parchment paper from the back of the computer screen and meter reader stickers. Place them on the front of the box.

8 Affix the button stickers and one of the black strips to the front of the box. Then take one of the 1.25-cm (½-in) wide black duct tape strips and cut it into 1.25 cm (½ in) squares and affix them to the front of the box.

9 Take another 1.25-cm (½-in) wide black duct tape strip and cut from it a thinner strip 6.5 mm (¼ in) wide and 12.5 cm (5 in) long. Affix this inside the meter shape as a dial. Cut small strips of red duct tape about 2.5 cm (1 in) long and approximately 6.5 mm (¼ in) thick. Place these at the top of the meter reader as units of measurement.

10 Cut a 25.5 cm (10 in) strip of black duct tape and place it on top of a piece of baking paper. Cut it into a squiggly line, then remove the baking paper backing and affix it to the inside of the computer screen.

82. Ace Card

Materials

» White duct tape
» Red duct tape
» A corrugated cardboard box, flat, approximately 45.5 x 30.5 x 30.5 cm (18 x 12 x 12 in)
» Brown paper

Additional Tools

» White grease pencil

1 Cut the box along the seams to create two flat panels. Cover one side of one of these pieces with white duct tape.

2 To make a heart template, first fold a piece of brown paper in half vertically, then draw and cut out a half-heart shape 30.5 cm (12 in) high and 15.25 cm (6 in) wide, then unfold it.

3 Make a one-sided layered fabric from red duct tape, 30.5 cm (12 in) square and backed with baking paper. Trace the heart template onto the fabric and cut it out. Remove the parchment backing and affix the heart to the white tape-covered panel's centre.

4 Create a word processing document containing four letter 'A's, using a bold sans-serif font like Abadi, Futura or Gill Sans, and a point size of 290pt. Print it out and use it as a stencil.

5 Make another red, baking paper–backed, one-sided layered duct tape fabric 21.5 cm (8½ in) wide by 28 cm (11 in) high. Place the stencil on top and cut out the four letter 'A's.

6 Remove the backing from the 'A's and affix one to each of the white panel's corners.

7 Cover one side of the second box panel with red duct tape.

8 Cut a 42 cm (16½ in) strip of white duct tape, and fold it in half with its sticky sides facing to create an 21 cm (8¼ in) long double-sided strip. Attach the ends of this strip to the inner sides of both panels, a few inches inward from one top corner. Repeat this step to make a second shoulder strap on the opposite side.

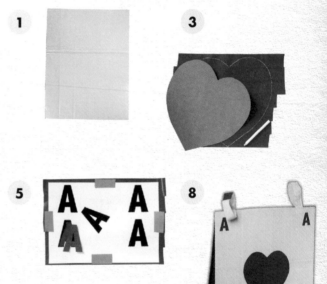

Materials

» Green duct tape

83. Grass Skirt

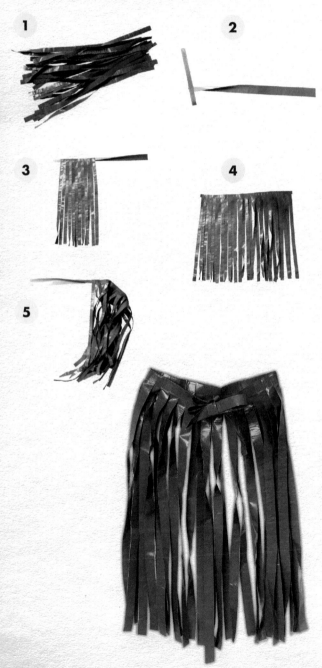

1 Cut a 61 cm (24 in) strip of green duct tape, then fold it in half lengthwise, with the sticky side facing inward. Repeat this step until you have twenty-eight of these strips, which will serve as the blades of grass.

2 Cut a 76 cm (30 in) strip of green duct tape. Fold it in half lengthwise, but with the sticky side facing outward this time. Hold the ends down with a metal ruler.

3 Starting on the left side, place the blades of grass on top of the duct tape strip, with each of them overlapping each other slightly.

4 When all the blades of grass have been placed, unfold the sticky strip and then refold it in the opposite direction, on top of the blades of grass. This forms the main part of the skirt.

5 To make ties at each end, attach strips of duct tape measuring at least 15.25 cm (6 in) to each end of the horizontal strip. Fold these strips in half lengthwise, with their sticky sides facing inward.

CHAPTER 9:

Seasonal

I love shopping for holiday décor. My usual routine consists of picking a day on the calendar to drive a few towns over to a well-stocked big box store and load up my car with lights, ornaments, banners or baskets. But what ultimately happens is this: I didn't get enough. Or I didn't buy the right colour. Or something breaks while in transit, and when I go back to return it I discover that the store has sold out of my precious trinket. Rats!

To compensate for any undesirable situation I may find myself in, I have turned to duct tape. Oh, yes. Duct tape holiday décor has saved me from a flavourless home, jazzing up an otherwise bland staircase or barren fireplace mantel. Each of the projects in this section has a proven track record in my own home.

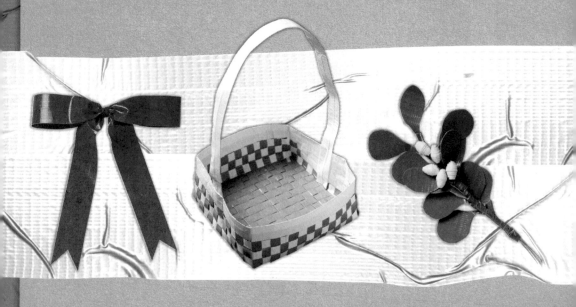

Materials

» Gold chrome duct tape
» Brown paper

84. Hanging Tree Ornament

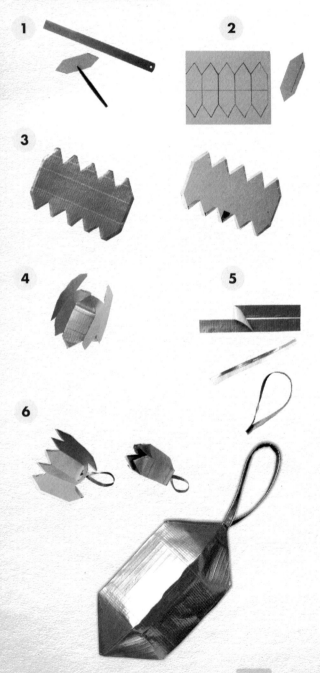

1 Draw a hexagonal stencil on brown paper. First, draw a rectangle 3.75 cm (1½ in) wide and 6.25 cm (2½ in) high, then draw two triangles extending 3.75 cm (1½ in) long from the rectangle's top and bottom edges.

2 On a larger piece of brown paper, trace the hexagonal stencil five times side by side, making sure to align the points.

3 Cut out this shape and cover it with strips of gold duct tape.
Cut around the shape, leaving a 3 mm (⅛ in) duct tape border. Fold these edges over on the shape's left sides only.

4 With the shape's gold side facing outward, bend the top points over inward, and seal their sides together with the open edges of duct tape until only one border is left unsealed.

5 Cut a 19-cm (7½-in) long strip of duct tape, halve it lengthwise, then fold this over three times, sticky sides facing inward, into a narrow strip, then fold into a loop.

6 Use small strips of duct tape to adhere the loop's ends to the inside of the ornament, and then to seal the ornament's remaining open sides, leaving the loop protruding from the top.

85. Candy Cane Ornament

1 Cut a 30.5 cm (12 in) strip of white duct tape, and lay it down sticky-side-up.

2 Cut a 61 cm (24 in) piece of steel wire. Fold it in half and place it on top of the white duct tape strip, then roll the white duct tape over the steel wire to form a thin stick.

3 Cut a 40.5 cm (16 in) strip of red duct tape, then cut a 6.5 mm (¼ in) wide strip from it. Use the red strips to add a spiral stripe around the white duct tape stick.

4 Bend the top of the stick over to form a cane shape.

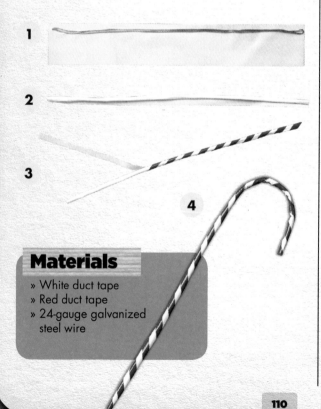

1

2

3

4

Materials

» White duct tape
» Red duct tape
» 24-gauge galvanized steel wire

Materials

» Red duct tape

86. Decorative Red Bow

1 Using the duct tape, make a double-sided layered fabric 61 cm (24 in) wide by 5 cm (2 in) high. Square up the sides.

2 Cut five strips measuring 5 mm (¼ in) wide by 5 cm (2 in) high. Pinch and fold the centre of the fabric. Hold in place with a small strip of duct tape. Set aside.

3 Make a second double-sided layered fabric measuring 61 cm (24 in) wide by 5 cm (2 in) high. Square up the sides. Pinch and fold the centre of the fabric, and hold it in place with a small strip of duct tape.

4 Place this second fabric on top of the first, aligning the pinched centres, and attach both pieces with a small strip of duct tape. Pull the ends of the second fabric down.

5 Take the ends of the first fabric and bring them to the middle. Pinch and fold the ends, then attach them to the centre with small strips of duct tape.

6 Cut triangular indents into the ends of the bow's legs and wrap one 1.25 cm (½ in) wide strip of red duct tape around the centre of the bow.

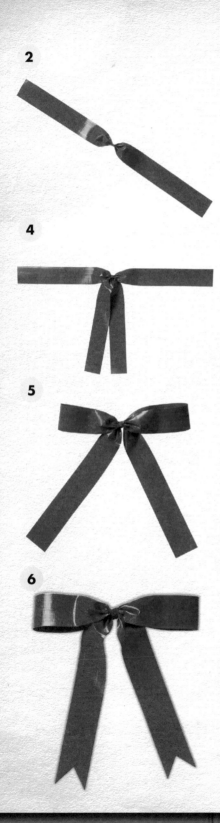

Materials

» 24-gauge galvanized
   steel wire
» Green duct tape
» Silver chrome duct tape

87. Mini Wreath

1 Cut a 71 cm (28 in) strip of green duct tape. Flip it over so the sticky side faces upward.

2 Cut a 71 cm (28 in) piece of steel wire, and place it lengthwise along the centre of the duct tape strip.

3 Place another 71 cm (28 in) strip of green duct tape over the first strip. Try to match up the edges as much as possible.

4 Using detail scissors, cut slits into both sides of the strip, avoiding cutting into the wire in the middle.

5 Repeat Steps 1 to 4 using silver chrome duct tape instead of green. Take the two strips and twist them together at least eight times. Attach the ends together with small strips of duct tape and fluff out the sides.

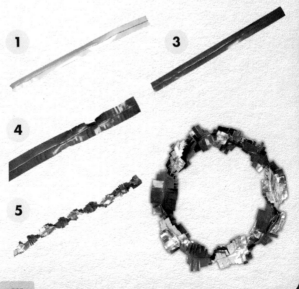

88. Stocking

Materials

» Red duct tape
» Green duct tape
» White duct tape
» Silver chrome duct tape
» Brown paper

Additional Tools

» White grease pencil

1 Draw and cut out a 38 cm (15 in) high stocking shape onto brown paper, with the top edge 19 cm (7½ in) wide and bottom edge 38 cm (15 in) wide.

2 Make two 41 cm (16 in) square double-sided layered duct tape fabrics. The first should have a green front side and white reverse side, and the second a red front side with a white reverse.

3 With the red side of the first fabric facing downward, place the first fabric directly on top with its green side facing upward; use small strips of tape to hold them in place. Trace the template onto the green fabric with a white grease pencil, then cut it out of both fabrics.

4 Cut a 41 cm (16 in) strip of silver chrome duct tape, then halve it lengthwise. With the two fabric pieces still aligned on top of each other, use one of the silver strips to close the stocking's seam down the long straight side.

5 Use the second strip to close up the seam on the opposite side. To seal the stocking's curved edges, cut slits into the silver tape on the outer side of the curve so that it can bend to follow it.

6 Cut another 23-cm (9-in) long strip of silver duct tape, halve it lengthwise, and use one half to seal the stocking's bottom seam.

7 Fold the remaining silver chrome strip in half lengthwise, sticky sides facing inward. Fold this in half into a 11.5 cm (4½ in) loop.

8 Use small strips of silver duct tape to attach the loop to the upper back edge of the stocking's opening.

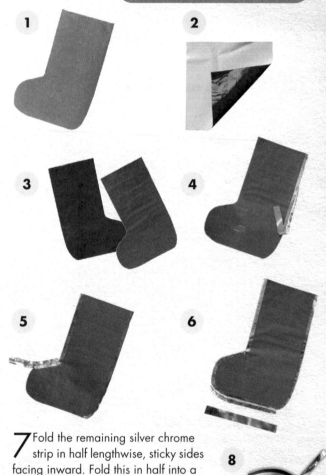

89. Mistletoe

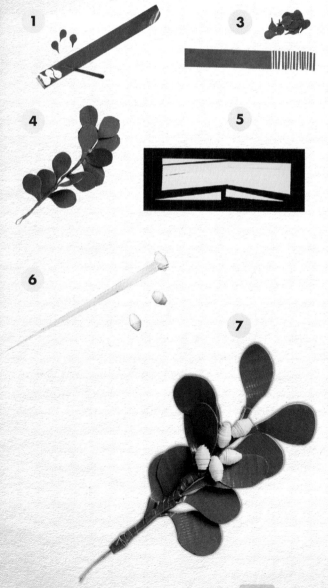

Materials

» Green duct tape
» White duct tape
» 24-gauge galvanized steel wire
» Mini glue dots

1 Cut two 41 cm (16 in) strips of green duct tape and combine them into a single double-sided strip. Use a craft knife to cut out twenty teardrop-shaped leaves, each of them 2 cm (¾ in) wide and 4.5 cm (1¾ in) long.

2 Cut a 30 cm (12 in) piece of steel wire and fold it in half.

3 Cut a 30 cm (12 in) strip of green duct tape then cut it into 6.5-mm (¼-in) wide strips.

4 Use these strips to attach each of the leaves to the steel wire at the stem. Cut another strip of green duct tape measuring 15–18 cm (6–7 in) long, then cut it lengthwise to make a 6.5-mm (¼-in) wide strip. Use this strip to cover the wire, weaving it around the attached leaves.

5 Cut an 20.5 cm (8 in) strip of white duct tape, then cut it lengthwise into 1.25-cm (½-in) wide strips. Cut each 1.25 cm (½ in) strip diagonally in half to create at least six long triangular pieces.

6 Roll the triangular pieces into beads, starting at their wider ends and finishing at their apexes. These are the berries of the mistletoe.

7 Attach the berries to the mistletoe with glue dots, arranging them in a cluster.

90. Spring Banner

1 Make a one-sided, 53.5 cm (21 in) square layered fabric from electric blue duct tape, and square up its sides.

2 Pull up the fabric and lay it on the cutting mat sticky-side-up. Affix the bandanna over the surface, smoothing out any air bubbles by hand. Flip over so that the blue duct tape side is facing up. This is the banner's background.

3 Make a green one-sided layered duct tape fabric measuring 56 cm (22 in) wide and three strips high. From the upper left corner cut a curved downward slope ending at the bottom centre. Pull up this sloped shape and affix it to the lower left corner of the banner.

4 Starting from the upper right corner of the green duct tape fabric, cut a downward slope ending at the bottom in the centre of the fabric. Pull up this slope shape and affix it to the lower right corner of the background.

5 Take the remaining piece of the green fabric and rotate it 180 degrees. Use the craft knife to round the top portion of the apex, then pull up the shape and affix it to the lower middle section of the banner, which should now feature three green hills.

Materials

- » Electric blue duct tape
- » Green duct tape
- » Lime green duct tape
- » Yellow duct tape
- » Orange duct tape
- » Brown duct tape
- » White duct tape

Additional Tools

- » Bandanna, at least 53.5 cm (21 in) square
- » Thin black marker

6 Make a white, one-sided layered duct tape fabric, 43 cm (17 in) wide and three strips high. Cut out two cloud shapes and affix them to the top of the banner.

7 Make a one-sided layered yellow duct tape fabric on top of baking paper, measuring 56 cm (22 in) wide and three strips high. Use the inner side of a duct tape to trace three circles onto the fabric, then trace three smaller circles with 3.75 cm (1½ in) diameters onto the same fabric. Cut out all six circles.

8 Remove the circles' baking paper backing and assemble the shapes of three chicks on the banner's green hills. Use the large circles as the chicks' bodies, and the small ones as their heads.

9 Cut out three teardrop shapes from the yellow duct tape fabric, each 2.5–4 cm (1–1½ in) wide and 5 cm (2 in) high. These are the chick's wings: add one to the side of each chick.

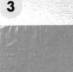

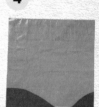
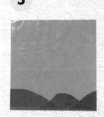
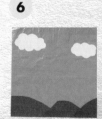

7

8

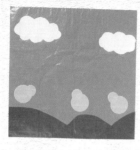

11

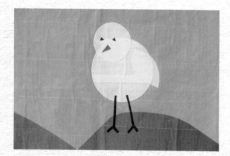

13

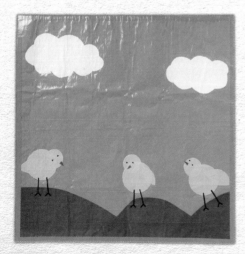

10 Cut out two small triangles from a small strip of orange duct tape strip. These are the baby chicks' beaks – add one beak to each chick.

11 Cut three pairs of legs and feet from a small strip of brown duct tape. Each leg should be 3 mm (⅛ in) wide and 3.75 cm (1½ in) high. Each foot should consist of two small strips 3 mm (⅛ in) wide and 1.25 cm (½ in) high. Affix a pair of legs and feet to each chick. Then, from the same brown strip of tape, cut out three pairs of triangular eyes, each 3 mm (⅛ in) wide. Add one pair of eyes to the faces of each chick.

12 If you would like to add text to the banner, use a word processing application such as Microsoft Word to create a text document containing the word or words you want to add. Use a plain modern font such as Abadi, Futura or Gill Sans, sized at approximately 220pt. Print out the document in the landscape position, then place it on top of a one-sided layered fabric (lime green would work well in this project) large enough to contain all of the text. Cut out the letters from the fabric, then affix the letters to the banner between the clouds and the chicks.

13 Cut two strips of lime green duct tape, each 56 cm (22 in) long, and cut them in half lengthwise. Add these strips to the edges of the banner as a border, and trim any excess tape.

91. Easter Basket

Materials

» 24-gauge galvanized steel wire
» Putty duct tape
» White duct tape

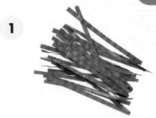

1 Cut a 56 cm (22 in) strip of putty duct tape. Cut it in half lengthwise, then fold each strip in half lengthwise with the sticky sides facing each other. Repeat this step until there are thirteen strips. Cut the strips in half so there are twenty-six strips measuring 28 cm (11 in) long.

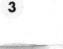

2 Weave the strips together, twelve on the vertical edge and fourteen on the horizontal edge. Leave space around the woven square, which should measure approximately 16.5 cm (6½ in). Be sure to push the strips together for a tight weave.

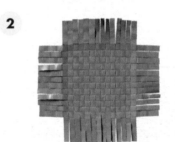

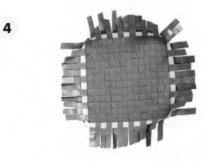

3 Cut two 69-cm (27-in) long strips of white duct tape, and halve them lengthwise. Fold three of these strips in half lengthwise, sticky sides facing inward.

4 Weave a white strip round the perimeter of the woven square. At each corner, pull up the next piece so that the sides begin to bend at 90-degree angles. Hold the corners together with small pieces of duct tape that can be removed later. When you get all the way round, seal the white strip with a small piece of white duct tape cut from the fourth strip, and trim off any excess.

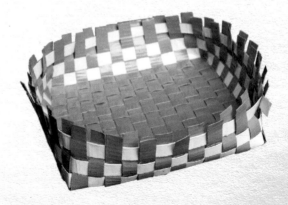

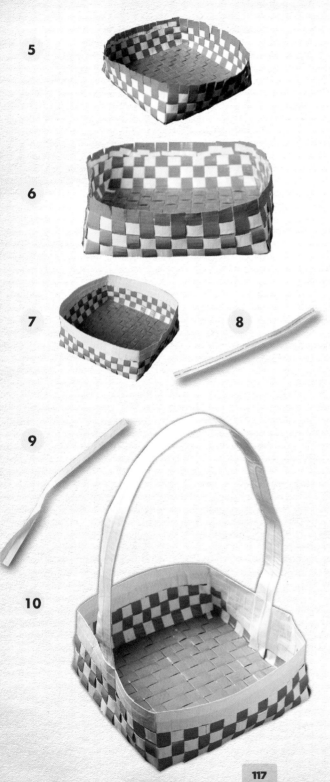

5 Weave in two more duct tape strips and tape the ends together once each of them has circled the perimeter. The square basket shape should now be able to hold its form.

6 On the inside of the basket, push the white strips together. Add small strips of white duct tape to the top of the upper white duct tape strip on the inside of the basket.

7 Trim off any excess putty-coloured strips around the top perimeter of the basket, so the sides are 5 cm (2 in) high on all sides. Then cut a 69 cm (27 in) strip of white duct tape and fold it over the top edge of the basket to an even horizontal mark all the way round.

8 Cut a 61 cm (24 in) strip of white duct tape. Fold in half lengthwise, sticky side facing inward. Place a 61 cm (24 in) piece of steel wire down the centre of the strip. Hold in place with small pieces of duct tape.

9 Cut a second 61 cm (24 in) strip of white duct tape. Place the first strip on top, lining up along one edge. Fold the strip over and cover the wire. This is the basket handle.

10 Curve the handle into a loop shape. Attach its ends to the inside of the basket, in the middle of two opposing sides, with strips of white duct tape.

CHAPTER 10:

Miscellaneous Projects

There is no end to the many uses that duct tape can be put to – it can be employed in a huge variety of crafty situations. From faux feathers that can be worn in your hair to a superhero cape for a Hallowe'en costume, duct tape has proven to be a versatile raw material. It makes sense to always have a roll or two tucked away in a drawer, 'just in case…'

The projects in this section remind me of a really good jambalaya I once ate. It was delicious, but what the heck was in it? After badgering the chef for the ingredients, he finally relented with a shrug of his shoulders and this nugget of non-commitment: 'A little of this, a little of that'.

This section contains projects that are book-related, repair-related and clothes-related. But is there any underlying theme to tie it together? Nah. It's a little of this, a little of that, and the jambalaya is quite tasty.

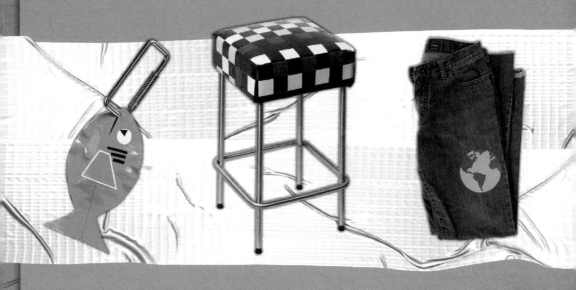

Materials

» Transparent duct tape
» Baking paper

92. Repairing a Book Cover

1

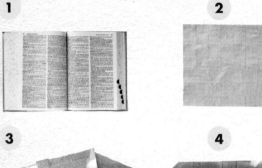

2

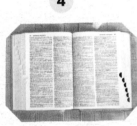

3

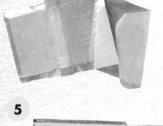

4

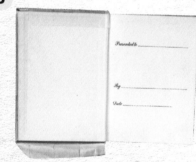

5

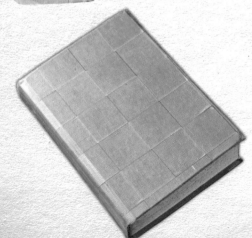

1 Place the book on top of the cutting mat. Open it so it lays flat on its spine. Measure the width and height of the open cover. Set the book aside.

2 Make a single-sided woven duct tape fabric on top of a piece of baking paper, measuring 5 cm (2 in) more than the book in both width and height. Square up the sides.

3 Open the book and place it on top of cutting mat with the cover facing up. Remove the parchment paper from the back of the woven fabric and, starting from the left edge, carefully roll the fabric onto the cover. Be sure to leave a 2.5 cm (1 in) fabric border around the perimeter of the book. At the top edge cut two slits into the border to indicate the width of the spine. Repeat at the bottom edge.

4 Remove the book cover's four corners, cutting them off at a 45-degree angle. The middle of the cut should just touch the corner of the book.

5 Fold in the borders over the inside of the front and back covers. Trim off the border pieces at the top and bottom edges near the spine.

93. Guitar Strap

1 Make a double-sided layered fabric 61 cm (34 in) wide by 6 cm (2½ in) high, with its front side red-and-yellow tie-dye and its reverse side yellow. Lay the fabric across the cutting mat at a 45-degree angle.

2 At one end, add a double-sided layered fabric 11.5 cm (4½ in) long (its front side black and reverse side gold) as an extension of the original fabric. Fold the tip of this extension in half lengthwise and use scissors to round the corners.

3 Unfold the extension. Use a hole puncher to cut a hole along the crease 1.25 cm (½ in) inward from the edge. Cut four small, 3-mm 9⅛-in) long slits inside the hole. This is the hole for the bottom of the guitar.

4 At the other end of the strap, add another black and gold, double-sided layered extension fabric, 5 cm (2 in) long.

5 Fold the tip of this extension in half lengthwise. Along the bottom edge, measure and mark 1 cm (⅜ in) from the folded corner. Cut the corner off at a 45-degree angle from this mark.

6 Cut two 51 cm (20 in) strips of black duct tape and fold each into thirds lengthwise, sticky sides facing inward. Combine them to create one 102-cm (40-in) long rope.

Materials

» Red and yellow tie-dye duct tape
» Yellow duct tape
» Black duct tape
» Gold chrome duct tape
» Velcro® strip (one side 30.5 cm (12 in) long, the other 8 cm (3 in) long)

Additional Tools

» 3 mm (⅛ in) hole puncher

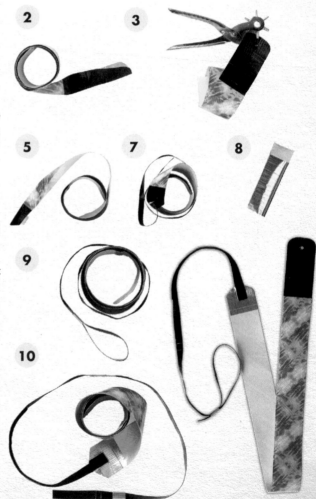

7 Cut a 2.5 cm (1 in) slit at approximately 1.25 cm (½ in) from the top edge of the top of the strap. Slip one end of the rope through the slit, and cover this end of the rope with a piece of black duct tape to hold it in place. Flip the strap over and cover the reverse side with gold chrome duct tape.

8 Cut a 7.5 cm (3 in) strip of gold chrome duct tape. On the upper left corner remove a rectangular piece measuring 1.25 cm (½ in) wide by 2.5 cm (1 in) high, and fold it in half lengthwise. You should have a double-sided strip measuring 5 cm (2 in) wide, with a 2.5 cm (1 in) sticky extension.

9 Double up the black duct tape rope in one hand. Wrap the gold duct tape strip around the rope. It should have a little bit of room to move up and down the length of the ropes. Press down on the sticky extension, forming a band. Pull out the end of the rope so it is not doubled up anymore within the gold band.

10 Flip the rope so that the reverse side is facing up. (The yellow side of the strap should be facing up, too.) Remove the backing of the 30.5 cm (12 in) half of the Velcro® strip. Place it on the rope near the base, where is connects to the main body of the strap. Then, remove the backing of the 7.5 cm (3 in) half of the Velcro® strip and place it on the tip of the rope.

94. Fixing the Hem on a Trouser Leg or Skirt

1 Adjust the hem of the trouser leg or skirt to desired height. Hold in place with straight pins.

2 Heat up the iron. Once it is at the appropriate temperature, place the iron over the hem to crease the fabric. Once the crease is made, turn off the iron and set it aside.

3 Remove the straight pins. Cut strips of duct tape and fix the hem in place with the tape from the inside.

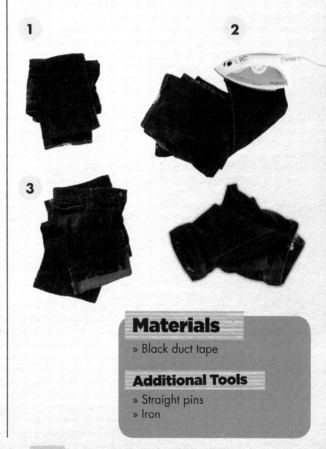

Materials
» Black duct tape

Additional Tools
» Straight pins
» Iron

95. Luggage Tag

Materials

» Pixilated camouflage duct tape
» White paper measuring 7.5 cm (3 in) wide by 4 cm (1½ in) high

Additional Tools

» Thin black marker
» Self-adhesive laminating sheet
» Glue dots
» Tweezers

1 On a rectangular piece of white paper, write down your name, address and telephone number. Remove the backing from a self-adhesive laminating sheet and smooth the adhesive side over the white paper, then trim the excess laminating sheet to leave a 6 mm (¼ in) sticky border.

2 Make a camouflage, one-sided layered duct tape fabric 15 cm (6 in) wide by two strips high. Place the fabric on the cutting mat sticky-side-up, then place the laminated white paper on top of the fabric, directly in the middle.

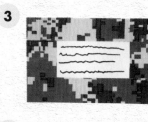 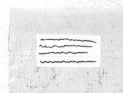

3 Place four strips of tape around the perimeter of the white paper, forming a rectangular frame around it. Measure 2.5 cm (1 in) from the outer edges of the white paper and trim off excess duct tape. This completes the body of the luggage tag – it should measure 13 cm (5 in) wide by 9 cm (3½ in) high.

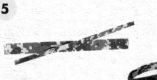 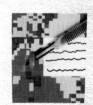

4 Measure and mark 1.25 cm (½ in) inward from the tag's left edge. Cut a 1.25-cm (½-in) long vertical slit along this mark, then cut two more 1.25 cm (½ in) slits next to it, each 3 mm (⅛ in) apart. Use tweezers to part these slits so that they are ready to weave through in Step 6.

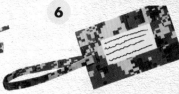 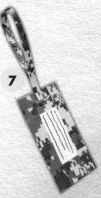

5 Cut a 30.5 cm (12 in) strip of duct tape and halve it lengthwise. Fold one of the strips in half lengthwise, sticky sides facing inward, into a short cord.

6 Weave the cord through the slits made in Step 4. Use a small piece of duct tape to attach the two loose ends of the cord together, forming a loop.

7 Near the cord's base, where it meets the tag, add a glue dot between the two sections of the cord. Press them together so that the tag stays flat.

Materials

» Leopard print duct tape

96. Wild Head-Phone Cord

1 Cut an 45.5-cm (18-in) long strip of leopard print duct tape, and cut the strip in half lengthways.

2 Place the headphone cord along the long edge of one tape strip and wrap it around the cord.

3 Repeat Step 2 with the second strip of tape, slightly overlapping the first covered length of cord. Repeat Steps 1 and 2 until the whole length of headphone cord is covered.

2

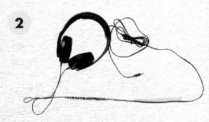

3

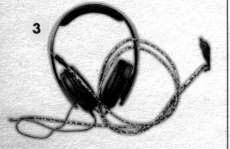

1

97. Bookmark

1 Cut two 15-cm (6-in) long strips of duct tape – one flame patterned, the other yellow – and affix them together, sticky sides facing.

2

2 Affix a 4-in (10-cm) long strip of orange duct tape to a piece of baking paper. Write your chosen word onto it in thick lettering, and cut out each letter. Remove the baking paper backing from each letter and affix them to the bookmark's hot rod side.

3

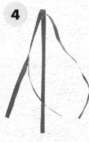

3 Fold the bookmark vertically in half, and cut round its top and bottom corners with a craft knife to round them off.

4 Cut a 30.5 cm (12 in) strip of orange duct tape, then halve it lengthwise. Fold one half in half again lengthwise, sticky side inward. Halve this lengthwise and bend each resultant strip in half. These will form tassels.

4

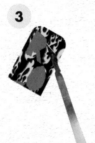

5 Use the hole punch to cut a hole through the top of the bookmark, push the folded ends of the tassel through and tie a single knot near the base. Trim the tassels' ends to make them even.

5

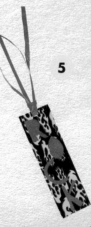

Materials

» Hot rod flame pattern duct tape
» Orange duct tape
» Yellow duct tape
» Baking paper
» 6 mm (¼ in) hole puncher

98. Book Cover

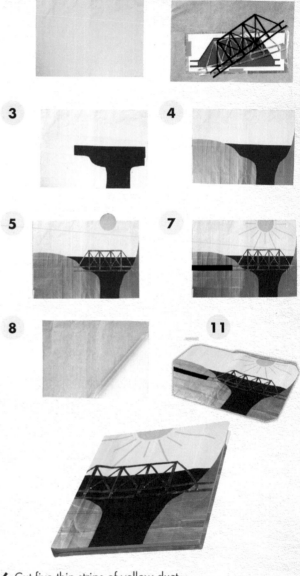

1 Make a white, one-sided layered duct tape fabric on top of baking paper, 48 cm (19 in) wide by 34 cm (13½ in) high.

2 Make a one-sided layered fabric from silver chrome duct tape, also on top of baking paper, measuring 38 cm (15 in) wide by 13 cm (5 in) high. Make a trestle bridge stencil (see page 51) 30.5 cm (12 in) long and 9.5 cm (3¾ in) high and place it on top of the fabric, securing it with masking tape along the edges. Cut around the stencil to make a silver trestle bridge sticker.

3 Make a one-sided fabric with blue duct tape with a top edge 32 cm (12½ in) wide, but which narrows to around 13 cm (5 in) at the bottom edge. This is the water. Place this shape on the lower right side of the cover.

4 Make a one-sided silver duct tape fabric 36 cm (14 in) wide by 22 cm (8½ in) high. Cut it into two curved shapes to form either side of a gorge, and affix them to either side of the water.

5 Remove the backing from the trestle bridge sticker and affix it to the cover between the two landmasses. Trace the inside circle of a duct tape roll onto a piece of yellow duct tape, cut it out, and place it overlapping the cover's top edge, toward its right side.

6 Cut five thin strips of yellow duct tape 3 mm (⅛ in) wide and 5 cm (2 in) long, then four more yellow strips 3 mm (⅛ in) wide and 9 cm (3½ in) long. Arrange these round the sun as sunrays, alternating between the long and short strips.

Materials

» White duct tape
» Deep ocean blue duct tape
» Silver duct tape
» Silver chrome duct tape
» Black duct tape
» Yellow duct tape
» Baking paper

Additional Tools

» Masking tape

7 Affix a 2.5 cm (1 in) wide strip of black duct tape running horizontally from the bridge's left edge to the cover's left edge.

8 Remove the backing from the cover and place it on the cutting mat, sticky-side-up.

9 Place the front of your book face-down on top of the left side of the book cover about 2.5 cm (1 in) from the left edge, with the book's spine on the right. Wrap the right side of the cover over the book, then smooth out any air bubbles by hand along the spine and back of the book.

10 Lay the book open on the cutting mat. Trim any excess cover around the book's edges down to a 2.5 cm (1 in) border. Cut two vertical slits into the border's top and bottom edges, in line with the edges of the spine. Cut off all four corners of the book cover at a 45-degree angle. The middle of each cut should touch each corner of the book.

11 Fold the borders over the book's edges onto the inside of the book's front and back covers. Trim off the border pieces at the top and bottom edges near the spine.

99. Patch for Ripped Denim Jeans

1

2

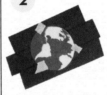

1 Cut out an illustration from a newspaper or magazine to use as a stencil (or use one of the examples on page 51) and separate out which shapes you want to appear as different colours.

2 Make a one-sided layered duct tape fabric on top of baking paper which loosely match the colours of your illustration. Place the illustration on top and hold in place with masking tape. Cut out the shapes in your chosen colours using a craft knife.

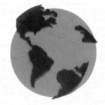

3 Place the pair of jeans on the cutting mat. Smooth out the area of the rip, trying to reassemble the original shape of the jeans.

4 Remove the baking paper backing from the sticker and place it on top of the rip. Smooth out any wrinkles.

To create the Planet Earth sticker, see the instructions on page 51.

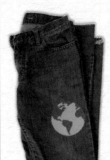

Materials

» Green duct tape
» Blue duct tape (or choose your own colours)
» Newspaper or magazine
» Baking paper
» Masking tape

100. Fish Key Chain

Materials

» Teal duct tape
» White duct tape
» Black duct tape
» Scrap paper
» Baking paper
» Fibrefill
» Key chain ring

Additional Tools

» 3 mm (⅛ in) hole puncher
» Thin black marker

1 Make a fish-shaped template on scrap paper measuring 8.25 cm (3¼ in) wide by 4.5 cm (1¾ in) high.

2 Cut a 13-cm (5-in) long strip of teal duct tape and place it on top of a piece of baking paper. Cut a second 13 cm (5 in) strip and place it on top of the first, overlapping by 6 mm (¼ in). Trace the template onto the tape with a black marker, then cut out the shape. Repeat this step to make another, identical panel.

3 Remove the baking paper from the one panel and place it on the cutting mat sticky-side-up. Roll a cotton-ball-size portion of fibrefill in your hand, and place it on the panel.

4 Remove the baking paper from the front panel and place it sticky-side-down on top of the back panel. Press the panels together round the edges.

5 Use a hole puncher to cut a hole near the shape's front tip.

6 Cut a circle from white duct tape with a 1.25 cm (½ in) diameter. This is the fish's eye – affix it to its head, then add a small triangle of black duct tape as the pupil. Cut a strip of black duct tape 1.5 mm (¹⁄₁₆ in) wide and 1.25 cm (½ in) long. Affix one strip below and in front of the eye as the fish's mouth.

7 Cut three more black duct tape strips, each 3 mm (⅛ in) wide and 1.25 cm (½ in) long, to use as gills. Affix these behind the fish's eye.

8 Cut a trapezoid from teal duct tape 2 cm (¾ in) wide on its bottom edge, 8 mm (⅓ in) wide at the top, and 2 cm (¾ in) high. Place it on top of a small piece of white duct tape and trim round it to create a 1.5-mm (¹⁄₁₆-in) wide white border. This is the fin – place it sideways in the centre of the fish.

9 Add the key chain ring through the hole.

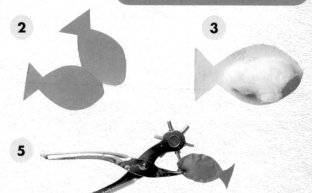

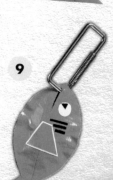

PROPERTY OF MERTHYR
TYDFIL PUBLIC LIBRARIES

Materials

» Brown paper
» Black duct tape
» Green duct tape
» White duct tape
» Silver duct tape

Additional Tools

» White grease pencil

101.
Reupholstering a Bar Stool

1 Place the brown paper on top of the stool. With the white grease pencil, trace the outline of the shape of the top side of the seat. This will be the seat cover's template.

2 Measure the depth of the seat. On the cutting template measure and mark the depth of the seat by extending the outer edges; add an additional 2.5 cm (1 in) border beyond this. Remove any excess paper from the border.

3 Make a woven duct tape fabric on top of a piece of baking paper. Randomly mix the colours, and ensure that the fabric is large enough to fit the cutting template inside it. Trim the woven fabric to the size of the seat template.

4 Remove the baking paper from the back of the fabric and cover the stool seat. Pinch the excess fabric at the corners and trim with scissors. Smooth down the sides and fold the edges of the fabric underneath the seat.

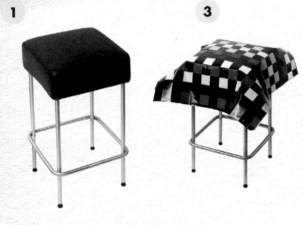

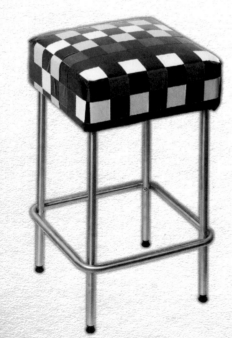

Online Resources

General Materials:
Uline, www.uline.com

General Art and Craft Supplies:
A. I. Friedman, www.aifriedman.com
Amazon, www.amazon.com
Dick Blick Art Materials, www.dickblick.com
Jerry's Artarama, www.jerrysartarama.com
Michaels, www.michaels.com
Pearl Fine Art Supplies, www.pearlpaint.com
Utrecht Art Supplies, www.utrechtart.com

Trimming:
M&J Trimming, www.mjtrim.com
Trim Fabric, www.trimfabric.com

Sewing and Quilting Supplies:
Home-Sew Inc., www.homesew.com
Sew True, www.sewtrue.com

Duct Tape Brands and Manufacturers:
3M, www.3m.com
Duck Brand, www.duckbrand.com
Nashua, www.nashua.com

Hair Accessories:
Factory Direct Craft, www.factorydirectcraft.com

Acknowledgements

The beginning of this book can be traced to the moment when someone posed a not-so-simple question to me: can you conceive – and write – 101 duct tape crafts? Sonya Ellis of Quintet Publishing asked the question that begat these projects. Sonya: thank you for fishing me out from the bottom of a barrel!

The making of a book involves many collaborators. For *Tape It & Make It*, most of them were the talented and driven individuals of the Quintet Publishing family. Editorial director Donna Gregory is one such individual, as is my editor Ross Fulton who happens to be part cheerleader, part cruise director and part machine. Ross: thank you from the bottom of my heart.

Over the years I've had the pleasure of making duct tape crafts with some crafty girls that are more precious to me than gold: Juliet Webb, Shea Betten, Sasha Reist, Grayson Liptack and my daughter Masana Morgan. Masana: you are everywhere – sometimes literally – in this book.

To my husband Dave and son Mack: thanks for all your patience while I stayed up writing and making a racket in my studio. You deserve homemade pizza for a month!

I have sisters and 'sisters' who constantly exhibit an open mind and critique everything I do with honest yet positive words: Elleanore Waka, Chonaliza Illonardo, Susan Lauzau, Hallie Einhorn and TD. Thank you for being in my life.